THE 5-INGREDIENT PALEO COOKBOOK

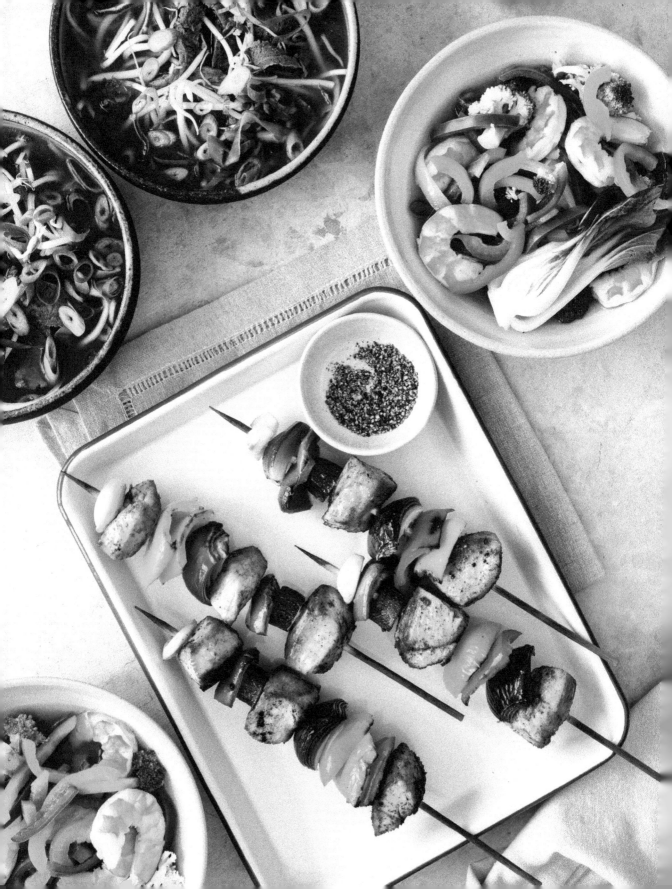

THE
5-INGREDIENT
PALEO
COOKBOOK

100+ EASY RECIPES for BUSY PEOPLE on the PALEO DIET

Genevieve Jerome

PHOTOGRAPHY BY NADINE GREEFF

ROCKRIDGE
PRESS

Interior and Cover Designer: Katy Brown
Photo Art Director: Amy Burditt
Editor: Brian Hurley
Production Editor: Andrew Yackira
Photography © Nadine Greeff, 2018

ISBN: Print 978-1-64152-111-6 | eBook 978-1-64152-112-3

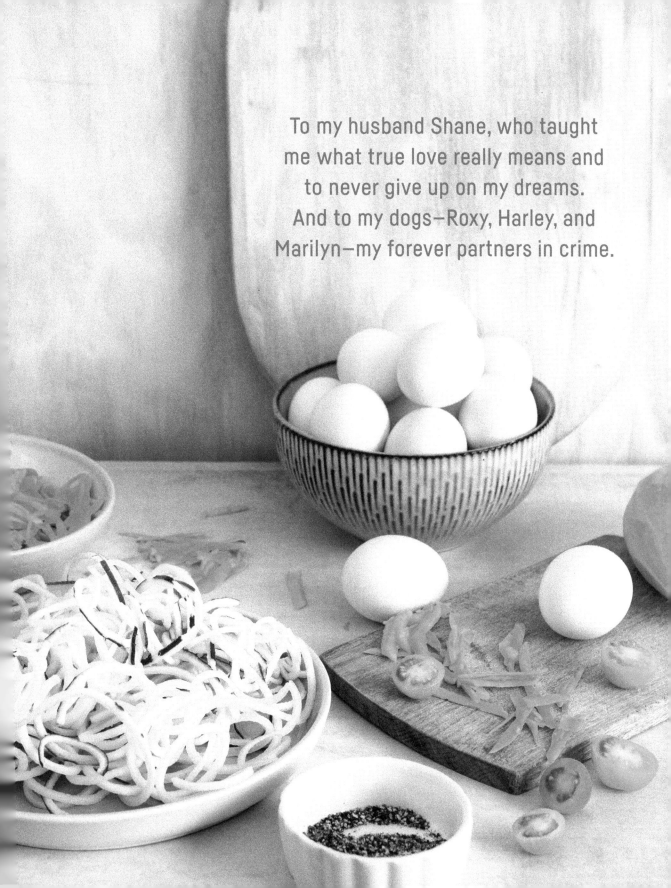

To my husband Shane, who taught me what true love really means and to never give up on my dreams. And to my dogs—Roxy, Harley, and Marilyn—my forever partners in crime.

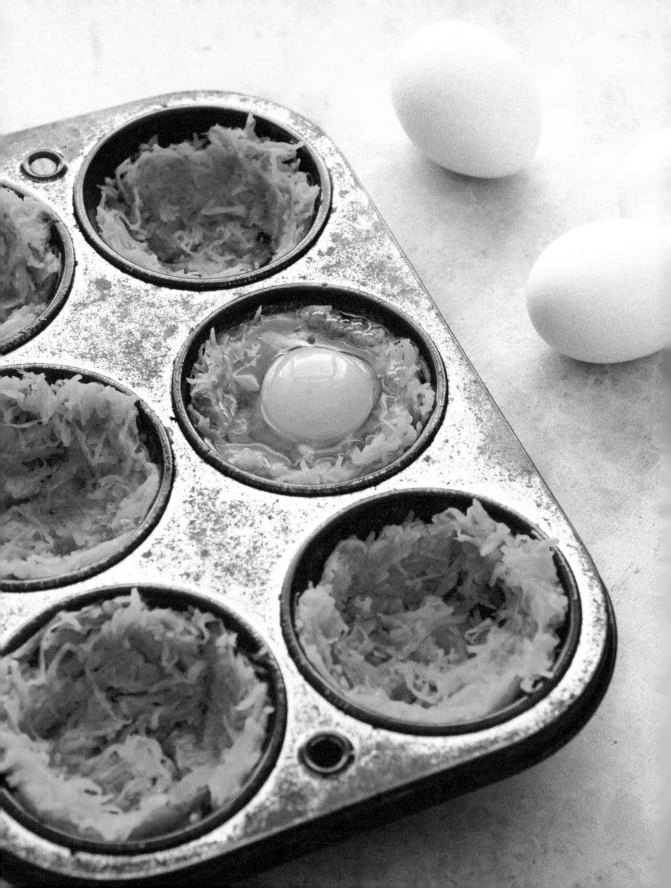

CONTENTS

INTRODUCTION

In 2011 I weighed nearly 280 pounds and was unhappy and constantly lethargic. I felt like there was a heavy weight not only on my body, but on my emotions, too. I felt worthless and I tried to eat my feelings. I used food as an escape rather than a refuge. I had no idea of the damage I was doing to my body. I thought eating when I felt down was the answer to my problems.

Then my doctor told me that, if I kept it up, my life could take a severely dark turn. So I walked out of her office, took her warning to heart, and started running that night. I worked out twice a day, starting with interval running. I would run for five minutes, then walk for five minutes, until I could run for thirty minutes a day without stopping.

Next, I looked at my food choices and realized something had to give. I stopped eating processed foods, cut out all sugar and sodas, and switched to sparkling water and regular water. I drank only black coffee, instead of sweetened coffee drinks, and ate all the veggies, potatoes, and fruit my body would allow. I googled trendy diets and found the Paleo diet. Doing that search saved my life.

The Paleo diet has allowed me to lead a healthy, active life. I'm proud to report I've successfully lost 155 pounds naturally through diet and exercise. And I'm always full of energy. It's a lifestyle, not a diet!

My life did a complete 180. I started my own business. I started my blog, *Fitty Foodlicious*, in 2016. Now, I'm a recipe and content creator—I write about health and wellness and how we can heal our bodies with food. I truly believe that if we eat the right foods and exercise every day, we can cure nearly anything that's ailing us—all while balancing our hormones at the same time. I also write about mental health and how our diet dictates our anxiety and happiness levels every day.

Adopting the Paleo lifestyle isn't easy, but it's completely adaptable. With *The 5-Ingredient Paleo Cookbook*, I have taken the fuss and complication out of cooking Paleo to give you simple, affordable, healthy recipes for you and your family. These are recipes you can come back to again and again. Many of them use only one cooking vessel. I am here to simplify your cooking!

Every ingredient in this book is natural, wholesome, and affordable, so you don't have to worry about what you are putting into your body. You will also save money by cooking these recipes because you won't have to eat at restaurants often. I've also listed ways to swap out certain ingredients, so this book works with nearly all food intolerances and allergies.

I hope you find solace and longevity in this cookbook. I hope you will learn to love the Paleo lifestyle as much as I do. I hope you will share this cookbook with your family and friends. I hope it brings you a lifetime of joy and many wonderful days of cooking healthy meals!

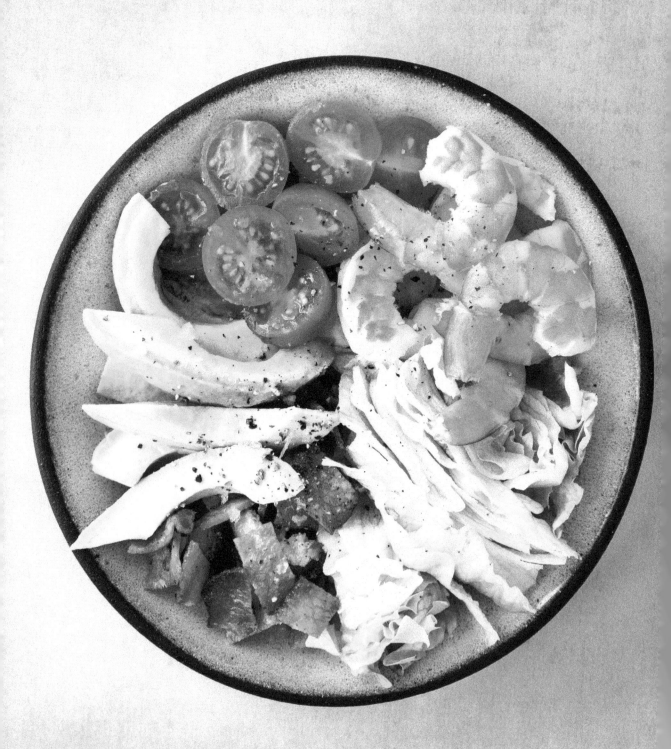

1

Simple & Easy Paleo Cooking

Life runs at warp speed these days and, when it comes to cooking and eating, healthy habits usually fall short. We make quick decisions and opt for unhealthy choices when, in reality, eating bad food will do more harm for our bodies than good. That's why my *5-Ingredient Paleo Cookbook* can be the answer to your prayers. I've created easy-to-follow recipes with step-by-step instructions that will have you looking forward to cooking and being in the kitchen. You will go from wondering what to buy at the grocery store, to grocery shopping as a favorite activity. These recipes are fun and healthy and offer a simple spin on a diet that has been around since cavemen (and women!) walked this earth. Welcome to *The 5-Ingredient Paleo Cookbook*. Now, let's dive in!

Opposite: Shrimp, Bacon & Avocado Salad, page 46

PALEO DIET GUIDELINES

There are many benefits to eating Paleo, including weight loss, clearer skin, higher energy levels, a stronger immune system, stable blood glucose levels, leaner muscles and less body fat, and better sleep, as well as many detoxifying benefits. Eating a Paleo diet may also help with diabetes, certain thyroid conditions, autoimmune issues, adrenal fatigue, and many digestive issues. Follow the diet—which at its core means avoiding processed foods, cereal grains, dairy, and legumes—to achieve these benefits and more.

How the Paleo Diet Works

Did cavepeople really eat this way?

The Paleo diet is based on what our cave ancestors would have eaten in what is commonly referred to as the Paleolithic Era. The Paleo diet mimics the natural foods cavemen hunted, foraged, and ate. This includes meat, fish, nuts, leafy greens, vegetables, healthy fats, and seeds. Foods to avoid on the Paleo diet are processed foods, high-sodium foods, refined vegetable oils, dairy, legumes, and cereal grains as they can contribute to thyroid issues, high blood sugar levels, and weight gain.

The Paleo diet has become popular in recent years due to the prevalence of people managing gluten and wheat allergies. People want a diet they can stick to, but one that is also sustainable. Eating Paleo is a simple, processed foods–free way of eating. Paleo is more than a diet; it's a way of life.

The Rules of Eating Paleo

The Paleo diet has certain guidelines; once you get the hang of these, the plan is easy to follow.

A PALEO DIET SHOULD BE HIGH IN ANIMAL PROTEIN. Opt for *grass-fed, pasture-raised, or locally sourced animals* as often as possible and look for ethically raised protein sources if at all possible. Meat that comes from nonlocal sources is typically pumped with high amounts of additives such as soy and wheat. The animals are often also treated unfairly and kept in inhumane conditions.

A PALEO DIET SHOULD BE HIGH IN SATURATED FATS, SUCH AS COCONUT OIL, BUTTER, GHEE, AND ANIMAL FATS. Eating good fat is good for you! Healthy fats help maintain a healthy heart as well as a lower body fat percentage.

A PALEO DIET SHOULD HAVE GENEROUS AMOUNTS OF FRESH VEGETABLES. Organic is always best, but not always possible. Follow the Dirty Dozen™ guidelines (see page 142) when deciding whether to buy organic versus nonorganic veggies and fruits. For example you don't need to buy organic avocados or bananas because you aren't eating the skin, and cauliflower and broccoli are sprayed with fewer pesticides than other vegetables. However, always buy tomatoes and strawberries as organic because they are sprayed with the most pesticides. When choosing fruits, opt for low-sugar fruits that are high in antioxidants, such as fresh berries.

A PALEO DIET ELIMINATES ALL REFINED SUGARS, INCLUDING FRUIT JUICES, *EXCEPT* LEMON AND LIME. Refined sugar spikes your blood glucose levels, which we want to avoid. Eliminating refined sugars will help naturally balance your blood sugar levels.

A PALEO DIET ELIMINATES ALL DAIRY, *EXCEPT* BUTTER. High amounts of dairy can cause blood sugar spikes as well as many digestive issues.

AVOID STRESS AND OPT FOR EIGHT HOURS OF SLEEP WHENEVER POSSIBLE. Stress wreaks havoc on the body; we need sleep to balance our hormones and keep our cortisol levels from spiking throughout the day.

EXERCISE IS KEY! Lifting weights and working out has been shown to reduce osteoporosis, certain cancers, and excessive weight gain. Aim for at least 30 minutes of exercise each day.

The recipes in this book will help you lead a healthy, active lifestyle—less time meal planning and shopping means more time for that walk or workout. Each recipe adheres to the preceding dietary guidelines and will make living a Paleo life easier and fun. With fresh, simple ingredients in each recipe, I take the thinking out of cooking and the stress out of mealtime! Plus, who doesn't love eating colorful food?

MAKING PALEO COOKING EASY

Cooking at home can be affordable and fun! The number one way to succeed on the Paleo diet is to plan your meals at the beginning of each week and cook at home.

PALEO FOODS TO ENJOY

Foods to enjoy in moderation are fruits that are high in sugar. Berries are always a wonderful option because they are low in sugar and do not spike your blood sugar levels like other fruits do.

Keep your servings of high-sugar fruits to 1 cup or less per day. If you have a fruit craving, opt for berries! When you are craving butter, opt for ghee and/or coconut oil instead.

Foods to Enjoy Freely

FRUITS

Apples

Avocado

Bananas

Blackberries

Blueberries

Cantaloupe

Figs

Grapes

Lemons

Limes

Lychee

Mango

Oranges

Papaya

Peaches

Pineapple

Plums

Raspberries

Strawberries

Watermelon

VEGETABLES/ HERBS

Artichoke hearts

Asparagus

Beets

Broccoli

Brussels sprouts

Cabbage

Carrots

Cauliflower

Celery

Cilantro

Eggplant

Parsley

Peppers

Scallions

Spinach

Squash (all varieties)

Sweet Potatoes

Yams

Zucchini

MEATS

Beef: grass-fed steak (New York/ strip steak); ground

Bison

Buffalo

Chicken: breasts, thighs, legs, and wings

Lamb rack

Pork: bacon; tenderloin and chops

Turkey

Veal

Venison steaks

FISH/ SEAFOOD/ SHELLFISH

Bass

Clams

Crab

Crayfish

Halibut

Lobster

Mackerel

Oysters

Salmon

Sardines

Scallops

Shrimp

Tuna

NUTS/SEEDS

Almonds

Cashews

Chia seeds

Hazelnuts

Macadamia nuts

Pecans

Pine nuts

Pumpkin seeds

Sesame seeds

Sunflower seeds

Walnuts

OILS/FATS/ VINEGARS

Fats: ghee, grass-fed butter

Oils: avocado, coconut, macadamia nut, olive

Vinegars: apple cider, balsamic, white wine

FOODS TO AVOID

Alcohol

Artificial sweeteners

Candy

Dairy

Fruit juices

Grains

Legumes (all bean varieties)

Refined sugar

Soda

Simple 5-Ingredient Recipes

Every recipe in this book uses 5 main ingredients, not counting your basic kitchen staples such as salt, pepper, and cooking oils. Keep your kitchen well stocked with these basics (which are not counted as part of the 5 main ingredients).

- Almond-coconut milk
- Cooking oil (coconut oil, ghee, olive oil)
- Fresh lemons and limes (no need to buy organic, as you won't eat the rind)
- Freshly ground black pepper
- Garlic
- Sea salt

Meal Planning Basics

Meal prep saves you time and money, plus you won't have to worry about what to cook for dinner. Following are my meal prep tips and tricks to keep your Paleo life sailing smoothly.

WRITE A GROCERY LIST EVERY SUNDAY AND STICK TO IT! The easiest way to fall off track is by adding things you don't need to your shopping cart. Once your grocery list is written, don't deviate from it.

NEVER GROCERY SHOP WHEN HUNGRY! Have a snack before you head into the store or, better yet, go grocery shopping right after lunch so you won't buy unnecessary items.

COOK FOODS AT ONCE. Roast all your veggies for the week. Slice them and roast them in batches so they're ready to eat at every meal.

MASON JAR SALADS ARE LIFESAVERS! You can get a case of tall Mason jars from a super-store fairly inexpensively. Fill the bottom of a jar with a salad dressing made of apple cider vinegar and extra-virgin olive oil (EVOO). Add your leafy greens and veggies. Placing the veggies at the top keeps them from getting soggy. Make and store a few in the fridge on Sunday night and you've got salads for lunch for the next few days.

Cooking Tips and Tricks

STORE FRESH HERBS IN ICE CUBE TRAYS. Chop a bunch of fresh herbs and mix them with EVOO. Fill ice cube trays and freeze. You'll have chopped fresh herbs ready to go. Simply add the herb ice cube to the pan and cook.

CHOP FRESH VEGGIES AHEAD OF TIME. If you don't have time to cook them ahead, you can get the prep out of the way. Slice, store in airtight glass containers, and stash in the fridge until needed.

CONSIDER PURCHASING CERAMIC COOKING PANS. Ceramic pans are great for cooking eggs because the food doesn't stick to the pan and there are no chemicals that leech out while cooking. My favorite brand is GreenPan and it is available at some superstores.

DOUBLE UP! Want frittata three times in one week? Make two batches on Sunday. The easiest way to avoid cooking every night of the week is to make double batches of the foods you love. Frittata anyone?

BUY IN BULK! Warehouse supermarkets often have wonderful deals on organic produce, fruit, and meat, so stock up on those items—especially meat, as it can get pricey—and freeze them for later use.

FREEZE INGREDIENTS. Prep your sides and meats on Sunday. Chop and cook all your veggies and meat on Sunday and store them in airtight containers in the freezer for easy access throughout the week.

MAKE SMOOTHIE BAGS! Purchase frozen fruit and combine different fruits in zip-top bags—one for each day of the week. Need a smoothie for breakfast? Simply grab one of your premade smoothie bags from the freezer, pop it in the blender with some water, and blend. It's smoothie time!

MAKE SPICE BAGS. Chop 2 or 3 garlic cloves, an onion, and a bundle of fresh parsley. Place in a zip-top bag and add 1 teaspoon each of sea salt and pepper. Seal the bag, shake everything up, and stash in the fridge. These spice bags are easy to grab throughout the week and make cooking so much easier because you don't have to spend time chopping and adding spices to everything. Use a prepared spice bag in stir-fry recipes, soups, stews, and anything cooked in the slow cooker. Sauté the contents of the bag in 1 tablespoon of EVOO, coconut oil, or ghee.

All the recipes in this book are perfect for practicing these tips and tricks that can help simplify your life!

THE PALEO-FRIENDLY KITCHEN

It is essential to have a well-stocked kitchen with certain items and equipment. If you do not already have these items on hand, preparing your kitchen will be a small investment, but one you can spread out over time. And, instead of thinking of dollar signs, think about how much you are investing in your health. If you already have these in your kitchen, fantastic! You're ready to get started. Following are my favorite kitchen essentials and the ones I use frequently.

Essential Kitchen Equipment

Let's start with the must-have items. These are items you will use to make many of the meals in this book. Following these are the nice-to-have items, which will make your meal prep a little easier, but aren't necessary if you don't want to use them.

Must-Haves

- BLENDER: You will need a high-power blender for all your soups and smoothies. This can also work as a food processor. It's a two-for-one kind of deal.

- CUTTING BOARD: This is a kitchen staple that every kitchen needs. You may even want two—keeping a dedicated one for meats.

- MEASURING CUPS AND SPOONS: A set of proper measuring cups and measuring spoons is essential for accurate measurements and better recipe results.

- PANS: I recommend a cast iron skillet, 18-by-13-inch sheet pan, and various sizes of sauté pans.

- SLOW COOKER: Look for affordable slow cookers at some superstores.

Nice-to-Haves

- CERAMIC PANS: These are a worthy investment that help with nonstick cooking, but certainly are not required.

- ELECTRIC PRESSURE COOKER: These are great for cooking meals in one vessel, but can be a tad pricey. Look for deals online if you want to add one to your arsenal.

- FOOD PROCESSOR: A food processor is wonderful, but a blender can be used for making homemade dressings, sauces, soups, and various desserts, and can function like a food processor for many items.

- SHARP KNIFE SET: Every kitchen should have a sharp knife, but a good one can be costly. Look for sets during sales! A full chef's knife set is useful when cooking at home. Cuisinart makes affordable sets.

- TOASTER OVEN: This is nice to have for sweet potato toast and reheating frozen meals.

Pantry Essentials & Cooking Staples

All the recipes in this book use 5 main ingredients, *excluding* the following essential ingredients to keep stocked in your kitchen:

- Almond-coconut milk
- Cooking oil (coconut oil, ghee, olive oil)
- Fresh lemons and limes
- Freshly ground black pepper
- Garlic
- Sea salt

Essential Pantry Items

- Beef gelatin
- Black pepper, freshly ground
- Cayenne pepper
- Cinnamon, ground
- Coconut aminos
- Coconut flour
- Coconut, unsweetened and shredded
- Cumin, ground
- Garlic powder
- Honey
- Nutmeg, ground
- Oils: avocado, coconut, extra-virgin olive (EVOO)
- Sea salt
- Tuna, canned and low-mercury
- Vinegar: apple cider, balsamic, white wine

Paleo Perishables

- Almond-coconut milk
- Almonds
- Avocados
- Berries, such as strawberries, blueberries, raspberries, and blackberries
- Dates
- Eggs
- Fresh ginger
- Fresh turmeric root
- Leafy greens such as kale, Swiss chard, spinach, and arugula
- Lemons
- Limes
- Sweet potatoes

Favorite Brands

- BOB'S RED MILL makes wonderful gluten-free and organic flours. All their ingredients are clean and perfect for the Paleo lifestyle.

- KRAVE makes affordable and tasty protein bars and snacks made from ethical meat sources.

- THE NEW PRIMAL makes wonderful, ethically sourced meat snacks, like jerky and beef sticks—must-haves for any Paleo person on the go.

- NUTPODS are good options if you must have creamer in your coffee. They make dairy-free creamer with a hint of sweetness.

- PRIMAL KITCHEN makes wonderful Paleo diet–friendly mayonnaise, oils, dressings, and snacks.

- VITAL PROTEINS is my favorite collagen peptides and beef gelatin brand! Vital Proteins sources their collagen and gelatin from ethical animal sources and are always up-front about the ingredients in their products.

ABOUT THE RECIPES

Starting a new diet can be hard, but it can be even harder if the recipes are overly complicated and call for ingredients you don't normally use on a regular basis. Don't worry—the recipes in this cookbook are easy to follow and each recipe uses just 5 main ingredients. The majority use kitchen staple ingredients you probably already cook with! The other bonus is that most can be made in under 30 minutes. Most recipes serve 4 to 6 people. Why complicate a good thing? I've also labeled every single recipe in this book to help you choose based on your needs that day. Keep an eye out for the following recipe labels:

30 MINUTES OR FEWER: These meals can be made in 30 minutes or fewer and still keep you and your family full and happy!

EGG-FREE: These recipes do not include eggs or egg whites.

FREEZER FRIENDLY: These meals freeze and store well. Prep on a Sunday, freeze, and have meals ready for the week.

NUT-FREE: These recipes do not use nuts or coconut.

ONE POT: One-pot recipes are my favorite! They can be made in a single pot, pan, baking dish, or bowl and are simple to prepare. Easy!

SLOW COOKER: Slow cooker meals are wonderful, especially for our busy lives. These can be prepped, tossed in the slow cooker, and ready when you come home.

Some recipes also include the following dietary labels:

VEGETARIAN: These recipes do not use meat but may include dairy, eggs, and honey.

VEGAN: These recipes do not use meat or any animal by-products.

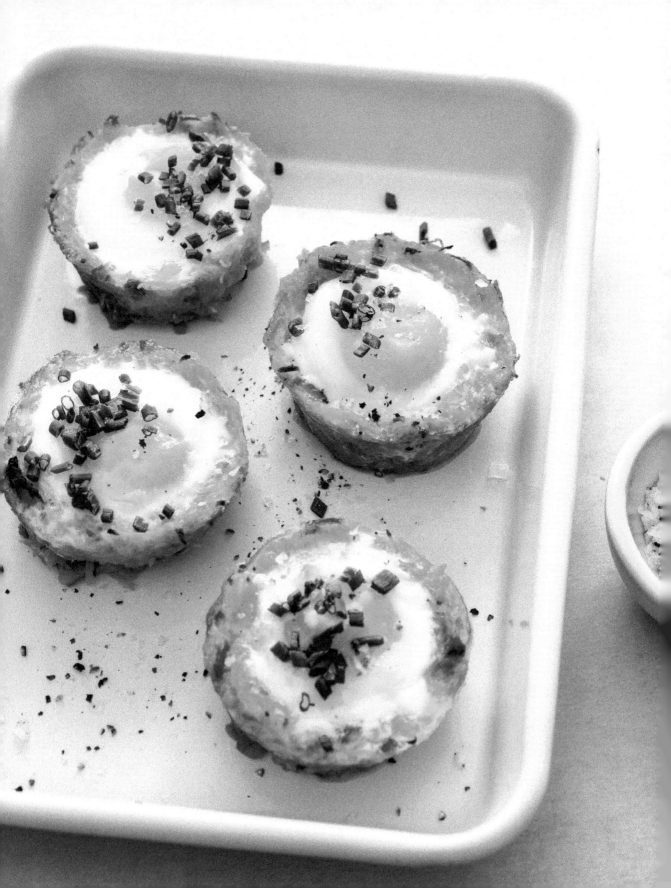

2

Smoothies & Breakfasts

Opposite: Sweet Potato Bird's Nests, page 26

Tropical Delight Smoothie

Prep time: 5 minutes / **Total time:** 10 minutes

This tropical smoothie makes a great post-workout snack and has the added bonus of making you feel like you're on a beach in Hawaii. One sip and you'll feel like you've been transported.

Smoothies are sometimes deemed unhealthy because they are often loaded with added sweeteners. They can actually be a great choice for easy and healthy meals on the go. When made with healthy ingredients—and without added sugar or other sweeteners—they provide ample vitamins and healthy fats. This one, for example, is loaded with vitamins B and C and healthy fats from the coconut and coconut milk. The coconut milk makes it a source of protein, and gives it a hint of sweetness as well.

Serves: 2 to 3

1 cup frozen cubed pineapple
1 cup frozen cubed mango
½ cup sliced orange
½ cup sliced guava
1 cup fresh almond-coconut milk
1 cup ice cubes
1 cup unsweetened shredded
   coconut, for topping (optional)
Pineapple slices, for
   garnishing (optional)

1. In a blender, combine the frozen pineapple, mango, orange, guava, almond-coconut milk, and ice. Blend on high speed for 2 to 3 minutes, or until nice and thick.

2. Pour the smoothie into a glass and top with shredded coconut and pineapple slices (if using). Add a paper umbrella for an extra dose of the tropics.

> **MAKE IT EASIER TIP:** Assemble all the ingredients at the beginning of the week and store in an airtight container. When you're ready for a smoothie, just put the prepped ingredients into a blender, blend, and you are ready to go. Yes, it's really that easy!

What's Left in the Fridge Smoothie

Prep time: 5 minutes / Total time: 10 minutes

I don't know about you, but I'm somewhat obsessed with cleaning and clearing out my fridge at the end of each week. I get the best feeling when my fridge is clean and fresh and I seriously feel like I can start my week on the right foot. Here's a way to do this and still use up the veggies and fruits on their way out—toss them in the blender and turn them into a delicious smoothie. You could use beets, apples, Swiss chard, and strawberries, or any combo you like. Use both fruit and veggies to keep your smoothie from tasting too bitter. Ever tried cauliflower in a smoothie? It's amazing! It makes your smoothie extra creamy and thick and makes it taste like rich ice cream, but without the calories. Whoever came up with the idea to add cauliflower to smoothies is a true genius in my book. You also get a nice protein boost in this smoothie with the help of collagen peptides (one of my favorite and easy ways to get protein).

Serves: 2 to 3

1 bunch fresh kale
½ head cauliflower, cut into florets
1 cup almond-coconut milk, divided
1 cup chopped nectarine
1 cup fresh strawberries, plus
   sliced strawberries, for
   garnishing (optional)
1 scoop collagen peptides
1 cup ice

1. In a blender, combine the kale, cauliflower, and ½ cup of almond-coconut milk. Blend.

2. Add the nectarine, strawberries, and remaining ½ cup of almond-coconut milk. Blend again on medium speed for 2 minutes.

3. Add the collagen peptides and ice. Blend on high speed until well combined. Serve in glass jars and garnish with additional strawberry slices (if using).

> VARIATION TIP: This smoothie is easy to adjust based on what you have in your fridge. Substitute spinach or other greens for the kale; peaches, plums, or apricots for the nectarine; and blackberries or blueberries for the strawberries.

Veggie Power Smoothie

Prep time: 5 minutes / **Total time:** 10 minutes

Find it hard to get your daily recommended allowance of veggies? Not to worry—this smoothie was made for you. With three servings of veggies, you could make this daily and be well on your way to getting your veggie fix. This smoothie is also loaded with fiber from the cruciferous veggies. It also has pectin from the apple, which aids the digestive tract in breaking down foods properly. Kale is hard on the digestive tract, but when blended in a smoothie it goes down easier and your body is able to process it better. Think of this recipe as a supplement, but one that comes from real food you can make any time of day.

Serves: 2

1 cup chopped kale
½ cup chopped broccoli
½ cup frozen cauliflower
1 cup chopped green apple, plus green apple slices, for garnishing (optional)
1 cup almond-coconut milk
1 tablespoon honey (optional)

1. In a blender, combine the kale, broccoli, cauliflower, chopped apple, and almond-coconut milk. Blend for 2 to 3 minutes until smooth and creamy.

2. Taste and add the honey (if using) for more sweetness, or omit it for a vegan version.

3. Pour into tall glasses and garnish each with an apple slice, if desired.

> **MAKE IT EASIER TIP:** Prep the ingredients at the beginning of the week and refrigerate in an airtight container. All you need to do is pour the prepped ingredients into a blender and you are ready to go! These can also be made into smoothie packs and stashed in the freezer.

> **PRO TIP:** Boil your veggies first, freeze them, and then add them to your smoothies. This helps your body absorb the nutrients from the veggies better and will help you digest everything.

Pumpkin Pie Smoothie

Prep time: 5 minutes / **Total time:** 10 minutes

I don't know about you, but once fall hits (well, let's be honest, July), I start thinking about pumpkin everything! And for good reason—it shows up everywhere, from lattes to loaf cake to pumpkin pie on Thanksgiving. It's easy to give in to temptation and eat all the sweetened pumpkin treats out there. But before you dive into pumpkin pandemonium, turn to this delicious and satisfying pumpkin smoothie instead. It uses honey, an all-natural sweetener, and is not overly sweet. Honey is processed in the body differently than refined white sugar. It takes a long time to break down and does not give you a sugar hangover later. It's an optimal sweetening source. This smoothie has a lovely, lightly sweetened pumpkin taste and a ton of fiber so it's a good, filling choice.

Serves: 2

1 cup canned pumpkin purée
½ cup pitted dates
2 scoops collagen peptides
1 tablespoon honey
1 cup almond-coconut milk
1 cup ice cubes
Ground cinnamon, for
    garnishing (optional)
Ground nutmeg, for
    garnishing (optional)

1. In a blender, combine the pumpkin and dates. Blend on high speed for 2 to 3 minutes.

2. Add the collagen peptides, honey, and almond-coconut milk. Blend again on high speed for 2 to 3 minutes.

3. Add the ice. Blend on high speed for 2 minutes more. Pour the smoothie into glasses and top with cinnamon and nutmeg (if using).

> MAKE IT EASIER TIP: Assemble the ingredients at the beginning of the week and freeze in airtight containers. All you need to do is pour the prepped ingredients into a blender and you are ready to go!

> VARIATION TIP: This pie-flavored smoothie is even more delicious when topped with coconut whipped cream.

Pineapple Mango Dreamin' Smoothie

Prep time: 5 minutes / **Total time:** 10 minutes

Got a fruity craving, but also need a protein kick? This smoothie will keep you strong on tough days. Mangos are wonderful because they are one of the sweetest fruits out there, but are also high in fiber and vitamin C. They are a very filling fruit, too, which makes this smoothie nice and robust.

Serves: 2

1 cup fresh or frozen chopped mango, plus fresh mango slices, for garnishing (optional)
1 cup fresh or frozen cubed pineapple, plus fresh pineapple slices, for garnishing (optional)
2 scoops collagen peptides
¾ cup pitted dates
1 cup almond-coconut milk
1 cup ice

1. In a blender, combine the chopped mango, cubed pineapple, and collagen peptides. Blend on medium speed until creamy. Add the dates and almond-coconut milk. Blend again.

2. Add the ice. Blend everything on high speed for 2 to 3 minutes until smooth. Pour the smoothie into glasses and garnish with fresh mango and fresh pineapple slices (if using).

VARIATION TIP: For an extra-creamy smoothie, combine the almond-coconut milk with the dates and collagen peptides and blend for 2 to 3 minutes until thickened, before adding the pineapple and mango.

Beets & Berries Smoothie

Prep time: 5 minutes / **Total time:** 10 minutes

Beets are very high in fiber, which is great for your digestive system. Half a cup of beets has 1.7 grams of fiber. This recipe contains that much beet per serving. Something to keep in mind regarding beets: They are red and may turn other things red, if you know what I mean. It's completely normal; what you see is just what your body hasn't absorbed. Berries are little nutritional powerhouses, with high doses of vitamin C and antioxidants to fight off free radicals. They help keep your skin clear and wrinkle free, and are essential to women's health. This high-fiber smoothie meets part of your recommended daily allowance of fruits and has electrolytes from the coconut water. This is a great smoothie to start your Monday.

Serves: 2

1 cup chopped raw beets
1 cup chopped kale
½ cup chopped banana
1 cup fresh or frozen blueberries, plus
    more for garnishing (optional)
1 cup coconut water
1 cup ice

1. In a blender, combine the beets, kale, and banana. Blend on low speed to mix.

2. Add the blueberries, coconut water, and ice. Blend on medium speed until smooth and creamy. Pour the smoothie into glasses and garnish with additional blueberries, if desired.

MAKE IT EASIER TIP: Assemble the ingredients at the beginning of the week and freeze in an airtight container. All you need to do is whiz the prepped ingredients in a blender and you are ready to go!

Vanilla Coconut Protein Smoothie

Prep time: 5 minutes / **Total time:** 10 minutes

This creamy vanilla smoothie with a hint of spice will remind you of childhood days eating ice cream, but without the high calorie count, and you get a nice protein boost from the coconut. Make this on a hot day and stay calm, cool, and collected. You could also add 1 cup of coffee to this smoothie to make it a morning wake-up call smoothie. You'll get extra energy, and a bunch of fiber, from the dates. And, did you know that cinnamon has been shown to prevent the spread of cancer cells? Organic ground cinnamon is best, but nonorganic cinnamon works, too. Cinnamon fights off the bad and helps keep the good in our bodies. I consume about 2 to 4 tablespoons of cinnamon per day and do my best to add it to everything—from coffee to smoothies to fruit. Cinnamon is truly the wonder spice! Vanilla is great for treating acne, improving hair growth, reducing inflammation, and preventing many chronic diseases.

Serves: 2 to 3

2 cups almond-coconut milk
1 cup pitted dates
1 tablespoon vanilla extract
1 tablespoon ground cinnamon, plus more for garnishing
1 cup frozen coconut chunks

1. In a blender, combine the almond-coconut milk and dates. Blend on high speed for 1 minute until smooth.

2. Add the vanilla, cinnamon, and frozen coconut chunks. Blend again for 1 minute until smooth and creamy.

3. Pour into glasses and garnish with a sprinkle of cinnamon.

> **VARIATION TIP:** For a different flavor, substitute almond extract for the vanilla.

Ham & Broccoli Egg Cups

Prep time: 5 minutes / Cook time: 35 minutes / Total time: 40 minutes

These ham and broccoli cups are the perfect breakfast on the go and are a fantastic source of protein. They also can be stored in the freezer in an airtight container for months. To reheat, warm 1 teaspoon of coconut oil in a skillet or ceramic pan over medium heat. Warm the egg cup for 2 to 4 minutes in the pan and enjoy!

Serves: 4 to 6

10 slices no-sugar-added ham
2 tablespoons coconut oil
½ cup chopped bell pepper,
   any color or a mix
1 cup chopped broccoli
½ cup almond-coconut milk
10 large eggs
Sea salt
Freshly ground black pepper

1. Preheat the oven to 375°F.

2. Line each well of a muffin tin with 1 slice of ham, forming a cup.

3. In a skillet over medium-high heat, melt the coconut oil. Add the bell pepper. Sauté for 3 minutes until softened.

4. Add the broccoli. Sauté for 5 minutes more until the broccoli begins to soften. Fill the ham cups about half full with the veggies, leaving room for the egg.

5. In a medium bowl, whisk the almond-coconut milk and eggs. Season with sea salt and pepper. Fill each muffin well to the top with the egg mixture. Using a toothpick, stir the veggies and egg together. This step is optional if you are looking for a more layered look to your egg cups.

6. Bake for 20 to 25 minutes until the eggs are set and the cups are slightly browned.

> VARIATION TIP: Substitute partially cooked bacon slices for the ham.

Paleo Breakfast Bowl

Prep time: 5 minutes / Cook time: 15 minutes / Total time: 20 minutes

This Paleo breakfast bowl is also great for lunch or dinner. It's packed with protein from the eggs and bacon. Get creative and substitute any Paleo-friendly toppings you desire. This recipe has one of my all-time favorite leafy greens: arugula. I'm obsessed with it. It's spicy, fresh, and vibrant. It perks up well when washed in cold water and lasts much longer than other leafy greens. It can be added to just about anything and tastes so good with some chopped bacon on top. All hail arugula!

Serves: 4

1 cup chopped uncooked bacon
2 cups arugula
1 cup cherry tomatoes
2 avocados, pitted and chopped
1 tablespoon coconut oil
4 large eggs
Sea salt
Freshly ground black pepper

1. In a skillet over medium heat, cook the bacon for about 5 minutes until crispy. Transfer to paper towels to drain and cool.

2. Divide the arugula among 4 serving bowls. Top each with cherry tomatoes, chopped bacon, and avocado chunks, placing them in different sections of the bowl.

3. Discard the grease in the skillet, wipe it out, and return it to medium heat. Add the coconut oil.

4. Carefully crack the eggs into the skillet. Fry until cooked to your desired doneness. You may need to fry one or two eggs at a time, depending on the size of your pan. Top each bowl with 1 fried egg, season with sea salt and pepper, and enjoy!

MAKE IT EASIER TIP: Make these salad bowls ahead of time by prepping all the veggies and dividing them among separate bowls. Cook the bacon and eggs on the day you want to eat the salad for breakfast!

Avocado Egg Cups

Prep time: 5 minutes / Cook time: 10 minutes / Total time: 15 minutes

These are a standard staple in any Paleo diet and are simple to make. Avocado egg cups are as popular on Pinterest as Birkenstocks in summer. That said, I created this recipe in 2006 when I got home from the gym one night and I was craving avocado and all its healthy fat. I like anything in a cup, so I came up with these avocado egg cups. These little guys are tasty and will keep you full for hours. Avocados contain the healthiest fats you can eat, which is why they appear so often in this cookbook. Also, no need to waste money on organic avocados as you are not eating the skin and, despite what some people believe, the pesticides do not leach into the thick skins of the avocados.

Serves: 4 to 6

3 avocados, halved lengthwise, pitted, and peeled
1 tablespoon freshly squeezed lemon juice
1 tablespoon coconut oil
6 large eggs
Sea salt
Freshly ground black pepper
1 cup fresh cilantro, finely chopped

1. In a medium bowl, toss the avocados in the lemon juice to keep them from turning brown.

2. In a skillet over medium heat, heat the coconut oil.

3. Carefully crack the eggs into the skillet. Fry until the whites are set. You may need to fry one or two eggs at a time, depending on the size of your pan. Season with sea salt and pepper. Carefully place each cooked egg into an avocado half.

4. Serve the avocado egg cups in ramekins, if desired. Top with cilantro and season again with sea salt and pepper, as desired.

VARIATION TIP: For a different take, you can bake the eggs right in the avocados instead of frying them. Just halve and pit the avocados (don't remove the peel) and scoop out some of the flesh to make room for an egg. Crack the egg into the hole, season with sea salt and pepper, and bake in a 425°F oven for 15 to 20 minutes until the egg is set.

Oven-Baked Omelets

Prep time: 10 minutes / **Cook time:** 25 minutes / **Total time:** 35 minutes

Omelets are a wonderful way to get started on your day's protein. This recipe can be made on a Sunday for the week, or stored in the freezer for months. It's versatile, has really good flavor, and will keep you satisfied for hours. Do you ever eat breakfast and then realize you are hungry two hours later? Me, too. That's because your breakfast is missing a key component, and that component is protein. Protein keeps you satiated throughout the day and prevents that awful sugar drop hours later—you know the one I'm talking about. With all the veggies, plus the eggs, you will feel good all day long.

Serves: 4 to 6

Nonstick cooking spray, for
  preparing the ramekins
8 large eggs
1½ cups almond-coconut milk
Sea salt
Freshly ground black pepper
2 cups chopped broccoli
2 cups fresh spinach
1 cup diced tomato
½ cup chopped fresh cilantro

1. Preheat the oven to 375°F. Coat 4 to 6 ramekins with cooking spray and set aside.

2. In a large bowl, whisk the eggs and almond-coconut milk until combined. Season with sea salt and pepper.

3. Add the broccoli, spinach, and tomato. Stir until well combined. Divide the egg mixture among the prepared ramekins.

4. Place the ramekins on a rimmed baking sheet and transfer to the oven. Bake for about 25 minutes until the eggs are no longer runny and the tops have browned a bit.

5. Serve garnished with fresh cilantro.

> **MAKE-AHEAD TIP:** Make a batch of these baked egg cups and stash them in the fridge or freezer. Pop them in the microwave to reheat, or just let them come to room temperature.

Sweet Potato, Ham & Egg Loaf

Prep time: 10 minutes / Cook time: 1 hour / Total time: 1 hour 10 minutes

This is an awesome freezer-friendly meal. It can be made on your prep day and frozen until needed. When following a Paleo diet, it is important to eat the entire egg. No egg whites only here! Dietary cholesterol from eggs does not raise your blood cholesterol. Egg yolks contain choline, essential B vitamins, and selenium, which our bodies need to function and metabolize foods properly. B vitamins are also essential to proper energy input. Don't fear the egg!

Serves: 4 to 6

2 tablespoons coconut oil
4 medium sweet potatoes,
    peeled and sliced
2 teaspoons paprika, plus
    more for the eggs
Sea salt
Freshly ground black pepper
1 medium red onion, sliced
2 cups chopped (½-inch cubes) ham
10 large eggs

1. Preheat the oven to 400°F. Line a 9-by-5-by-3-inch loaf pan with parchment paper. This keeps your loaf from sticking to the pan. Set aside.

2. In a skillet over medium heat, melt the coconut oil. Add the sliced sweet potatoes and season with the paprika, sea salt, and pepper. Sauté for 8 to 10 minutes. Add the red onion. Sauté everything for 5 minutes more.

3. Stir in the ham and sauté for 10 minutes. Transfer the sweet potato mixture to the prepared loaf pan.

4. In a large bowl, whisk the eggs. Season with paprika to taste. Slowly pour the eggs onto the sweet potato mixture. Bake for 25 to 30 minutes, or until the eggs are set and everything is nice and crispy.

5. Let cool for 5 minutes before slicing and serving.

VARIATION TIP: For added flavor and nutrition, add 1 cup chopped asparagus along with the ham.

Sheet Pan Breakfast

Prep time: 15 minutes / **Cook time:** 20 minutes / **Total time:** 35 minutes

Sheet pan breakfasts are easy and fast to make, and great for feeding a crowd. Sheet pan breakfasts are also a fantastic protein source and use minimal cookware. They are a popular Paleo staple because of the amount of food you can make at one time and the minimal cook time needed.

Serves: 4 to 6

Coconut oil spray, for preparing
  the sheet pan
1 cup chopped cauliflower
1 cup chopped broccoli
1 cup chopped bell pepper,
  any color or a mix
¼ cup EVOO
Sea salt
Freshly ground black pepper
2 cups ground sausage
4 to 6 large eggs (one per person)

1. Preheat the oven to 425°F. Coat a sheet pan with coconut oil spray and set aside.

2. In a large bowl, combine the cauliflower, broccoli, and bell pepper. Pour the EVOO over the veggies and stir to coat. Season with sea salt and pepper. Set the veggies aside.

3. In a skillet over medium heat, cook the sausage for about 5 minutes until just browned. Do not overcook; it will cook more in the oven. Add the veggies and stir to combine. Using a slotted spoon, transfer the sausage-veggie mixture to the sheet pan.

4. Make 4 to 6 holes in the mixture, one hole for each egg.

5. Bake the veggies and sausage for 10 minutes.

6. Remove the sheet pan from the oven. Carefully crack 1 egg into each hole.

7. Bake everything for 5 minutes more, or until the eggs whites are set.

> **SUBSTITUTION TIP:** Need a vegetarian option? Easy. Swap the meat for more veggies. Instead of sausage, use portobello mushrooms and asparagus.

Avocado Egg Sammies

Prep time: 5 minutes / Cook time: 10 minutes / Total time: 15 minutes

Breakfast sandwiches are one of my favorite morning meals because they are versatile, quick to prepare, and can easily be made with ingredients you have in your fridge. This recipe delivers your protein, veggies, and carb portions, plus a plethora of healthy fats. These sammies should keep you full for a while. Make them in batches and refrigerate in airtight containers for up to 3 days. If you don't want to use bacon, opt for sausage, Canadian bacon, or even thick slices of chicken. Avocados appear in nearly every main recipe in this book, and for good reason. They are versatile and count as one of the healthiest fats around. Avocados also make your hair grow and your nails nice and shiny.

Serves: 4 to 6

1 (12-ounce) package
  nitrate-free bacon
1 tablespoon ghee
4 to 6 large eggs
4 to 6 tablespoons Homemade
  Mayonnaise (page 126)
4 to 6 medium sweet potatoes, baked
  and halved (see preparation tip)
4 to 6 avocados, halved, pitted,
  peeled, and sliced

1. In a skillet over medium-high heat, cook the bacon for about 5 minutes, until crispy. Transfer to paper towels to drain and cool. Once cooled, halve each bacon slice widthwise.

2. In a clean skillet over medium-high heat, heat the ghee.

3. Carefully crack the eggs into the skillet. You may need to fry 1 or 2 eggs at a time, depending on the size of your pan. Fry until the whites are set.

4. Spread 1 tablespoon of mayonnaise on each sweet potato half.

5. Top each half with some avocado slices, bacon slices, and 1 fried egg.

6. Carefully top the egg with the other sweet potato half. You now have breakfast sammies!

PREPARATION TIP: Bake your potatoes beforehand in a 450°F oven for 45 minutes and then slice them in half.

VARIATION TIP: If you are vegetarian, swap the meat for a giant slice of portobello mushroom.

Sweet Potato Bird's Nests

Prep time: 10 minutes / Cook time: 30 minutes / Total time: 40 minutes

This is one of my favorite "make-ahead" recipes. You could easily prep part of this recipe the night before, and add the eggs the next morning to save time. This recipe is also great for kiddos because they can get creative with the bird's nests and add the toppings they want. Bird's nests are popular in the breakfast world, but I've put a Paleo spin on this breakfast tradition to make it accessible for people with specific dietary needs. We use shredded sweet potato hash to make the nests, and crack an egg in the middle for the protein. Sometimes, we like to top with chopped bell pepper and bacon bits for additional zest and flavor.

Serves: 4 to 6

Nonstick cooking spray, for
    preparing the muffin tin
4 medium sweet potatoes
1 tablespoon coconut oil
1 (12-ounce) package nitrate-
    free bacon, chopped
6 large eggs
4 tablespoons minced fresh chives
Sea salt
Freshly ground black pepper

1. Preheat the oven to 400°F. Coat a 6-cup muffin tin with cooking spray.

2. In a food processor fitted with the shredding blade, or a high-powered blender, finely shred the sweet potatoes. You could also use a spiralizer for this.

3. In a large skillet over medium-high heat, heat the coconut oil.

4. Add the shredded sweet potatoes and chopped bacon. Cook for 10 to 15 minutes until the sweet potatoes are softened and browned. Carefully scoop 2 to 3 tablespoons of the sweet potato mixture into each prepared muffin cup, pressing the mixture against the sides and bottom to form small nests, leaving room for the eggs.

5. Crack 1 egg into each nest.

6. Bake for 10 to 12 minutes, or until the eggs are no longer opaque. Let the nests cool for 2 to 3 minutes.

7. Once cooled, remove from the muffin tin, top with fresh chives, and season with sea salt and pepper.

> SUBSTITUTION TIP: If you want to make this vegetarian, omit the bacon and use shredded carrots instead.

Avocado Bacon Eggs Benedict

Prep time: 15 minutes / Cook time: 20 minutes / Total time: 35 minutes

This is one of my favorite twists on a breakfast classic. So many people freak out when they can't have bread anymore on the Paleo diet, because they think they can't have breakfast staples like eggs Benedict. But that is simply not true. This Benedict skips the carbs and high-fat hollandaise sauce. Instead, I use avocado-cilantro purée for the hollandaise.

Serves: 4 to 6

2 (12-ounce) packages
  nitrate-free bacon
4 to 6 avocados, peeled,
  halved, and pitted
1 cup fresh cilantro, minced,
  2 tablespoons reserved for serving
½ cup freshly squeezed lemon juice
2 tablespoons chopped garlic
½ cup EVOO
4 to 6 large eggs (1 per person)
Sea salt
Freshly ground black pepper

1. Preheat the oven to 400°F. Line a baking sheet with parchment paper.

2. Using about 5 bacon slices per egg, make them into a base. Lay the 5 pieces side by side on the prepared sheet, overlapping them slightly or weaving them if you feel ambitious. Bake for 15 minutes, or until crispy.

3. While the bacon cooks, in a food processor, combine the avocado, cilantro, lemon juice, garlic, and EVOO. Purée until smooth. Stash your avocado purée in the fridge to keep it cold until the eggs are done.

4. Bring a medium pot of water to a boil over high heat.

5. One at a time, crack an egg into a small bowl and slip it into the water. Cook until the whites have set, 2 to 4 minutes.

6. Place each bacon base on a plate. Using a large slotted spoon, gently remove the eggs from the water and top each base with 1 egg. Cover the eggs with avocado purée.

7. Sprinkle with the reserved cilantro and season with sea salt and pepper.

VARIATION TIP: For extra flavor, add a jalapeño pepper to the food processor along with the avocado. Remove the pepper's rib and seeds if you want just a little kick of spice.

Breakfast in a Jar

Prep time: 10 minutes / **Cook time:** 15 minutes / **Total time:** 25 minutes

Breakfast in a Mason jar is another favorite of mine. This recipe is easy to make and takes no time at all. All you do is prep and layer the ingredients into the jars. You can make them ahead, and they will keep in the fridge for up to 5 days. These handy little breakfast jars also travel well. Simply pop a top on the jar and you're good to go! These are a far better option than going through a drive-through somewhere, spending money you don't need to spend, and eating ingredients from who knows where.

Serves: 4 to 6

8 to 10 large eggs
2 cups almond-coconut milk
1 tablespoon ghee
1 pound ground turkey
Sea salt
Freshly ground black pepper
3 cups sliced mushrooms
3 cups shredded carrots
Minced fresh cilantro, for
   garnishing [optional]

1. In a large bowl, whisk the eggs and almond-coconut milk.

2. In a large skillet over medium heat, melt the ghee.

3. Add the eggs to the skillet and scramble to your desired doneness. Transfer to a bowl and set aside.

4. Return the skillet to medium heat and add the turkey. Season with sea salt and pepper. Cook for 4 to 6 minutes until browned. Transfer to a bowl and set aside.

5. Return the skillet to medium heat and add the mushrooms and carrots. Sauté for 3 to 4 minutes until thoroughly cooked.

6. Grab your Mason jars. Place a scoop of scrambled eggs in the bottom of each jar.

7. Add a layer of turkey followed by a layer of carrots and mushrooms. Repeat the layers until each Mason jar is almost full.

8. Garnish with fresh cilantro (if using) and season again with sea salt and pepper. These will keep, covered, in the fridge for up to 5 days. Serve warm or cold.

> **VARIATION TIP:** For an even more flavorful dish, add 2 minced garlic cloves along with the mushrooms and carrots.

Coconut Broccoli Frittata

Prep time: 10 minutes / **Cook time:** 40 minutes / **Total time:** 50 minutes

In the mood for a frittata? I have a unique and delicious recipe just for you—loaded with healthy fats and starring fresh coconut. Yes, you read that right. Fresh coconut!

I up the fiber game with broccoli, and your star protein sources are turkey and eggs. This is a winning meal! Want to make this vegetarian? Simply swap out the turkey and bacon for chopped kale and Swiss chard. You can get creative with this recipe and the best part is, it freezes really well. Thaw before reheating in a 250°F oven for 5 to 10 minutes. Just like that, breakfast is served!

Serves: 4 to 6

Coconut oil spray, for
    preparing the skillet
1 pound nitrate-free bacon
1 pound ground turkey (free-
    range if available)
2 cups almond-coconut milk
8 to 10 large eggs
4 cups chopped broccoli
4 cups unsweetened
    shredded coconut

1. Preheat the oven to 375°F.

2. Spray a cast iron skillet with coconut oil spray and place it over medium heat. Add the bacon. Cook for about 5 minutes until browned. Transfer to paper towels to drain and cool. Once cooled, chop the bacon into bits.

3. Wipe out the skillet and return it to medium heat. Add the turkey. Cook for 4 to 5 minutes until browned. Transfer to a bowl and set aside. Wipe out the skillet.

4. In a large bowl, whisk the almond-coconut milk and eggs.

5. Add the broccoli and coconut to the egg mixture. Whisk to combine. Slowly pour the egg-veggie mixture into the cast iron skillet. Top the egg-veggie mixture with the ground turkey. Top everything with the bacon bits.

6. Bake for 25 to 30 minutes, or until golden brown.

> **VARIATION TIP:** Feel free to substitute other veggies like halved cherry tomatoes, or chopped asparagus or kale.

Breakfast Salad

Prep time: 10 minutes / **Total time:** 10 minutes

Salad for breakfast? Don't knock it 'til you try it; once you do, I bet this will be a weekly breakfast staple in your household. And, this is probably one of the easiest breakfasts you can make in under 10 minutes. Let's dive into why this is a simple yet satisfying meal. You will easily get your recommended allowance of veggies in this meal with the leafy greens, bell peppers, and olives. You'll get a protein boost from the egg. Overall these breakfast salads are great to prep the night before. You only need to cook the eggs in the morning. Or, you can prep the hard-boiled eggs a few days before, as they will keep in an airtight container in the fridge for up to a week. This is also a great "I got invited to brunch last minute and have no idea what to make" recipe. You're welcome.

Serves: 4 to 6

6 cups fresh leafy greens
1 cup black olives
2 bell peppers, any color or a mix, diced
4 to 6 large hard-boiled eggs, peeled and sliced
Dressing of choice (see chapter 9), for serving

1. Place the greens in a large bowl. Add the black olives and bell peppers. Gently toss to combine.

2. Top the salad with egg slices.

3. Add the dressing and toss the salad to coat.

> **MAKE-AHEAD TIP:** To make these ahead on your food prep day, add the dry salad to Mason jars and top each with egg slices. Stash your dressing in a separate airtight container until ready to eat.

Baked Salmon & Lemony Kale Bowls

Prep time: 5 minutes / Cook time: 25 minutes / Total time: 30 minutes

Salmon is a wonderful protein source, especially for breakfast. It's loaded with omega-3s, healthy fats, and is a lean, clean protein. That said, purchase salmon from reputable sources. Don't go cheap here because farmed salmon is full of mercury and other toxic chemicals. Plus, it doesn't really taste that great. The ethically sourced kind tastes better, usually has more moisture, and cooks better, too. You want your salmon to be flaky and shiny once cooked. Be careful not to overcook the salmon, as it will dry out. Pair this dish with eggs and veggies and you've got one winning Paleo meal.

Serves: 4 to 6

Olive oil cooking spray, for
    preparing the baking dish
2 (6-ounce) salmon fillets
Sea salt
Freshly ground black pepper
1 tablespoon ghee
1 medium red onion, diced
1 bunch fresh kale, rinsed and chopped
1 cup freshly squeezed lemon juice

1. Preheat the oven to 400°F. Lightly coat a baking dish or sheet pan with cooking spray.

2. Season the salmon with a little sea salt and pepper. Place the salmon, skin-side down, in the prepared dish. Bake for 10 to 15 minutes, or until it's flaky but not dry. You don't need to flip the fish; it will cook just right in the oven.

3. Once the salmon is cooked, turn off the oven, but leave the fish inside until you are ready to slice it. Alternatively, remove it from the oven and cover with aluminum foil.

4. In a medium skillet over medium-low heat, heat the ghee. Add the red onion. Cook for about 5 minutes until brown.

5. Add the chopped kale. Sauté for 2 minutes.

6. Add the lemon juice. Sauté until the kale is bright green and the lemon juice has been absorbed.

7. Cut the cooked salmon into chunks.

8. Divide the kale among serving bowls and top with the salmon chunks.

MAKE-AHEAD TIP: Cook your veggies ahead of time and freeze in airtight containers, if necessary. When ready to eat, all you need to do is cook the salmon and warm the veggies.

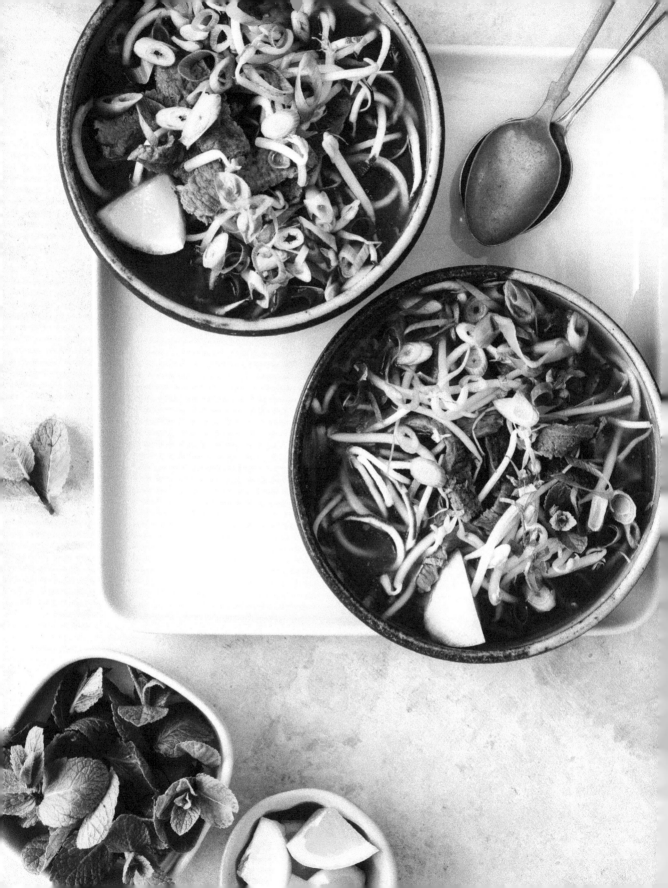

3

Hearty Soups & Salads

Opposite: Paleo Beef Pho, page 39

Butternut Squash Soup

Prep time: 20 minutes / **Cook time:** 50 minutes / **Total time:** 1 hour 10 minutes

This easy fall soup can be made any time of year. It will give you that cozy autumn feeling and it is hearty and delicious. It also freezes very well, where it will keep for up to 1 year (that's really planning ahead!). Bone broth is a great ingredient—packed with protein, vitamins, and tons of minerals. You can toss the butternut squash seeds or save them and roast for a yummy snack.

Serves: 4 to 6

1 (1- to 3-pound) butternut squash, halved lengthwise, seeds and pulp removed
3 tablespoons peeled and minced fresh ginger
¼ cup chopped red onion
1 cup almond-coconut milk
3 cups chicken bone broth
2 tablespoons ghee
Sea salt
Freshly ground black pepper
½ cup chopped fresh parsley (optional)

1. Preheat the oven to 350°F.

2. Place the squash halves, cut-side down, on a baking sheet. Bake for 45 minutes, or until the squash pierces easily with a fork. Remove from the oven and set aside to cool.

3. In a blender or food processor, combine the ginger, red onion, and almond-coconut milk. Using a spoon, scoop the cooled squash into the blender. Blend everything on medium-high speed until smooth. Transfer to a soup pot and place the pot over medium-high heat. Stir in the bone broth and ghee. Cook for 5 minutes.

4. Serve seasoned with sea salt and pepper and garnished with fresh parsley (if using). The soup will keep, refrigerated in an airtight container, for up to 3 days.

> **SUBSTITUTION TIP:** You can easily make this vegetarian. Just use vegetable broth or water in place of the chicken broth. To make it vegan, also substitute coconut oil for the ghee.

Slow Cooker Beef Stew

Prep time: 20 minutes / Cook time: 6 hours 5 minutes / Total time: 6 hours 25 minutes

This hearty beef stew will send you straight back to cold winter nights cozied up by the fire. It's a Paleo spin on the winter soup we all know and love. This slow cooker beef stew has tons of protein, freezes really well for later meals, and tastes rich, delicious, and full of flavor. It can be eaten with Cauliflower Tortillas (page 139) and makes wonderful leftovers. I recommend sprinkling chunky sea salt on this stew; it brings out the vibrant flavors of the dish and helps everything come together. This freezer-friendly dish will keep in the freezer, in an airtight container, for up to 6 months.

Serves: 4 to 6

2 pounds beef chuck roast, cubed
Sea salt
Freshly ground black pepper
6 cups beef stock
2 garlic cloves, chopped
1 medium white onion, diced
4 celery stalks, sliced
6 medium sweet potatoes, cubed

1. In a saucepan over medium heat, cook the beef for 4 to 5 minutes until cooked through. Transfer to the slow cooker and season with sea salt and pepper.

2. Add the beef stock, garlic, onion, and celery. Top with the sweet potatoes. Gently stir to combine. Cover the cooker and set to high heat. Cook for 6 hours.

3. Serve the stew garnished with more sea salt and pepper, as needed.

> VARIATION TIP: Add 2 sliced carrots and a few sprigs of fresh herbs, such as rosemary and thyme, to the dish along with the sweet potatoes.

> PRO TIP: You will need a slow cooker for this recipe; find one in a superstore or online.

Mexican Chicken Soup

Prep time: 20 minutes / **Cook time:** 35 minutes / **Total time:** 55 minutes

Do you ever crave salty soup? I know I do, especially on cold days. This delicious Paleo Mexican chicken soup will quell those salty cravings. The other nice thing about this recipe is that it also works as a cold soup in summer. This soup has robust flavors and a ton of nutritional benefits. You will get your protein boost from the chicken and all the healthy fats from the avocado. This recipe also freezes well and can easily be warmed on the stove for a quick bite. Top it with avocado and coconut cream and you'll have a dreamy soup and an easy go-to recipe.

Serves: 4 to 6

4 cups chicken stock
1 roast chicken, shredded
2 cups cauliflower rice
2 cups freshly squeezed lime juice
2 avocados, halved, pitted, and sliced
1 tablespoon full-fat coconut
    cream [optional]

1. In a large pot over medium heat, bring the chicken stock to a low simmer.

2. Add the shredded chicken and cauliflower rice. Simmer for 20 to 30 minutes until the soup starts to thicken.

3. Stir in the lime juice.

4. Serve the soup topped with avocado slices and coconut cream (if using).

> **VARIATION TIP:** Add a bunch of chopped fresh cilantro to the soup along with the lime juice.

> **MAKE IT EASIER TIP:** Buy a rotisserie chicken for this recipe so you don't have to spend hours cooking the chicken.

Roasted Cauliflower Bacon Soup

Prep time: 5 minutes / Cook time: 1 hour 40 minutes / Total time: 1 hour 45 minutes

This hearty soup is both delicious and filling. Cauliflower is quite big right now! It's on everyone's social media accounts and new cauliflower products are flooding the stores. It gets its good rep because it's hearty, rich tasting, and you can really do anything with cauliflower. It doesn't take long to cook either, which is another bonus. It's very popular for a reason! This freezer-friendly soup will keep frozen, in an airtight container, for up to 6 months, or in the fridge for up to 5 days.

Serves: 4 to 6

1 (12-ounce) package
   nitrate-free bacon
2 pounds cauliflower, cut into florets
4 cups chicken stock
2 cups full-fat coconut cream
4 garlic cloves, minced
Sea salt
Freshly ground black pepper

1. Preheat the oven to 425°F. Line a roasting pan with parchment paper and set aside.

2. In a skillet over medium-high heat, cook the bacon for about 5 minutes until crisp. Transfer to paper towels to drain. Chop the bacon and set aside.

3. Spread the cauliflower florets evenly in the prepared roasting pan. Roast for 20 minutes. Do not over-roast the cauliflower. You want it crispy, but not too brown.

4. Transfer the cauliflower to a large saucepan and place it over low heat. Add the chicken stock, coconut cream, and garlic. Simmer for 1 hour.

5. Add the chopped bacon. Simmer for 10 minutes more, or until thick and creamy.

6. Serve the soup seasoned with sea salt and pepper.

VARIATION TIP: Garnish with fresh herb sprigs, such as thyme or oregano.

Cream of Mushroom Soup

Prep time: 20 minutes / **Cook time:** 40 minutes / **Total time:** 1 hour

Cream of mushroom soup is a traditional soup recipe and a staple in American culture. I remember my grandmother cooking cream of mushroom soup many times throughout the years. It's delicious, creamy, and freezes well. This version is made with creamy coconut milk so it tastes rich, but it's really healthy. Mushrooms are nutritional powerhouses! Some people don't like their taste. I urge you to try this recipe, even if you don't like mushrooms, because of their amazing health benefits. This freezer-friendly soup will keep up to 1 year in the freezer.

Serves: 4 to 6

¼ cup ghee
1 medium red onion, chopped
2 garlic cloves, minced
4 cups sliced button mushrooms
4 thyme sprigs, stems removed,
  plus more for garnishing
4 cups vegetable stock
3 cups full-fat coconut cream, plus
  more for garnishing (optional)
Sea salt
Freshly ground black pepper

1. In a large pot over medium heat, melt the ghee.

2. Add the red onion and garlic. Sauté for about 7 minutes, until the onion is browned.

3. Add the mushrooms and stir to combine.

4. Add the thyme leaves. Cook for 2 minutes.

5. Pour in the vegetable stock and coconut cream. Bring to a simmer. Cook for 20 to 30 minutes until the soup is thick and creamy.

6. Serve garnished with more thyme leaves (if using) and seasoned with sea salt and pepper. You could also drizzle in some coconut cream, if you like.

> **SUBSTITUTION TIP:** Make this soup vegan by substituting coconut oil for the ghee.

Paleo Beef Pho

Prep time: 10 minutes / Cook time: 45 minutes / Total time: 55 minutes

Pho is having a major moment right now. Make my Paleo version and you won't need to spend money on the pricey restaurant version. My soup packs the protein and is low in sodium. The flank steak gives it a wonderful flavor without being overbearing. Plus, this Paleo pho will make you full. It's hearty, but lean. Buy a big batch of flank steak, slice it up, freeze it, and save it for the days you want to make this soup.

Serves: 4 to 6

4 cups beef stock

1 cup chopped fresh mint,
   2 tablespoons reserved
   for garnishing

1 cup chopped fresh basil,
   2 tablespoons reserved
   for garnishing

6 cups zucchini zoodles

1 pound flank steak, thinly sliced

6 lemon or lime wedges, for
   serving (optional)

1. In a medium pot over medium heat, bring the beef stock to a simmer.

2. Add the mint and basil. Simmer for 2 to 3 minutes.

3. Add the zucchini zoodles. Simmer for 30 minutes.

4. Add the flank steak. Simmer for 5 minutes more until the steak is just cooked through.

5. Serve the soup garnished with the reserved basil and mint. Serve garnished with lemon or lime wedges for diners to squeeze into their soup, if desired.

> PRO TIP: For the most tender meat, slice the steak thinly against the grain.

Asparagus Soup

Prep time: 15 minutes / **Cook time:** 30 minutes / **Total time:** 45 minutes

Asparagus soup is delicious, but many people often mistake it for pea soup. Instead of going for your traditional pea soup recipe, make this instead. Asparagus is one of my favorite veggies. We actually grow it on our farm and I'm pretty obsessed with the stuff. Asparagus has amazing health benefits, too. It's wonderful for your skin and heart, and has tons of vitamins. Make this easy soup any night of the week. Bonus: It freezes well, too!

Serves: 4 to 6

2 tablespoons EVOO
6 scallions, white and light green
   parts chopped, 2 tablespoons
   reserved for garnishing
3 pounds asparagus, woody ends
   removed and discarded, chopped
4 medium Russet potatoes,
   peeled and chopped
6 cups vegetable stock
4 cups full-fat coconut cream
Sea salt
Freshly ground black pepper

1. In a Dutch oven or large soup pot over medium heat, heat the EVOO.

2. Add the scallions. Sauté for 2 to 3 minutes.

3. Add the asparagus. Cook, stirring occasionally, for 5 minutes.

4. Add the potatoes and vegetable stock. Cover the pot. Bring to a simmer. Cook for 15 to 20 minutes until the potatoes and asparagus are soft.

5. Stir in the coconut cream. Using an immersion blender, purée the soup until smooth. Alternatively, transfer the soup to a blender (you may have to do this in batches) and purée until smooth. If you've used a blender, return the soup to the pot.

6. Bring the soup to a simmer again. Cook for 5 minutes until thick and creamy.

7. Garnish with the reserved scallions and season with sea salt and pepper.

> **VARIATION TIP:** Add 2 minced garlic cloves along with the scallions.

Radish & Cucumber Salad

Prep time: 10 minutes / Total time: 15 minutes

This is the easiest salad you will ever make and I'm willing to bet you already have the ingredients in your fridge. This classic salad will keep you cool on hot days and works as a refreshing side dish. It also makes a wonderful appetizer. The fresh dill makes the flavors pop even more, and it's colorful. I love colorful dishes! Make this when last-minute guests come over or when your parents surprise you!

Japanese cucumbers can be found any time of the year in many grocery stores. They are seedless and never bitter, which is why they make a wonderful ingredient in recipes.

Serves: 4 to 6

1 cup Homemade Mayonnaise
   (see page 126)
Sea salt
Freshly ground black pepper
4 Japanese cucumbers, thinly sliced
2 bunches radishes, thinly sliced
6 scallions, white and light
   green parts chopped
½ cup chopped fresh dill

1. Place the mayonnaise in a small bowl and season with sea salt and pepper. Stir to combine.

2. In another small bowl, combine the cucumbers, radishes, and scallions.

3. Pour the mayonnaise over the veggies and sprinkle the fresh dill over everything. Gently stir to combine and serve.

MAKE-AHEAD TIP: To help this recipe last longer, add 1 tablespoon of distilled white vinegar; the salad will last in the fridge, in an airtight glass container, for up to 1 week.

Tomato & Spinach Salad

Prep time: 10 minutes / **Total time:** 15 minutes

Another one of my favorite veggies (or fruits, depending on who you talk to) is the tomato. I adore tomatoes. When my hubby and I go out to a restaurant, I always ask him to give me his tomatoes. I LOVE them! This salad is refreshing, vibrant, and easy to make. Did you know tomatoes are loaded with lycopene? Our bodies need lycopene and, in fact, most Americans do not get enough. Well, this recipe gives you the recommended daily amount. Tomatoes also help keep your skin clear—make a refreshing facial mask using tomato juice, sea salt, and lemon juice. You're welcome. Enjoy this salad anytime of the year, but it's especially good in the warmer months.

Serves: 4 to 6

2 cups tricolor cherry tomatoes, halved
4 heirloom tomatoes,
    sliced ¼ inch thick
4 cups fresh baby spinach leaves
1 cup fresh basil leaves,
    coarsely chopped
1 cup EVOO
½ cup balsamic vinegar
Sea salt
Freshly ground black pepper

1. In a large bowl, combine the cherry and heirloom tomatoes.
2. Add the spinach and basil.
3. Drizzle with the EVOO and vinegar at once.
4. Sprinkle with sea salt and pepper, and serve.

> **INGREDIENT TIP:** It's perfectly fine to use wilted tomatoes for this recipe.

Avocado Cilantro Tuna Salad

Prep time: 15 minutes / **Total time:** 20 minutes

This tuna salad is full of healthy fats and protein and is packed with flavor. Tuna is a wonderful protein source, and very affordable. In this recipe, it pairs with vibrant cilantro and avocado. This salad can also be made ahead by prepping the veggie portion the night before and adding the tuna and dressing the morning of.

Serves: 4 to 6

½ cup freshly squeezed lemon juice
½ cup EVOO
Sea salt
Freshly ground black pepper
4 avocados, halved, pitted, and diced
2 cups mercury-free canned tuna
2 Japanese cucumbers, diced
1 medium red onion, sliced
1 bunch fresh cilantro, minced, plus
    leaves reserved for garnishing

1. In a medium bowl, combine the EVOO and lemon juice. Season with sea salt and pepper. Whisk to blend.

2. Add the avocados, tuna, cucumbers, red onion, and cilantro. Gently stir to combine. Serve garnished with cilantro leaves.

SUBSTITUTION TIP: Use canned wild-caught salmon in place of the tuna.

Cucumber & Carrot Salad

Prep time: 15 minutes / **Total time:** 20 minutes

You will need a spiralizer for this recipe. You can find one relatively affordable online. This is one of the easiest recipes you will ever make. Got carrots and cucumbers about to go bad? Not to worry—this recipe is perfect for those. The cucumbers in this recipe bring out the flavor of the carrots. The zesty dressing makes this the perfect refreshing meal.

Serves: 4 to 6

4 cucumbers, spiralized
4 carrots, spiralized
2 tablespoons pumpkin seeds, plus more for garnishing
1 cup chopped scallions white and light green parts
1 cup apple cider vinegar
1 cup freshly squeezed lime juice
1 cup EVOO
Sea salt
Freshly ground black pepper

1. In a large bowl, combine the spiralized cucumbers and carrots. Top with the pumpkin seeds and scallion.

2. In a medium bowl, whisk the vinegar, lime juice, and EVOO. Drizzle the dressing over the veggies. Season the salad with sea salt and pepper.

3. Serve garnished with pumpkin seeds.

> **VARIATION TIP:** Add chopped fresh cilantro leaves along with the scallion for even more flavor.

Taco Salad

Prep time: 5 minutes / Cook time: 10 minutes / Total time: 15 minutes

Craving tacos? This Paleo taco salad will make all those cravings disappear. It's loaded in flavor, has the veggie and protein combos your body needs, and has all the healthy fats from the avocado. I suggest using free-range grass-fed beef for this recipe. Organic grass-fed beef has better flavor and a lower fat content. This taco salad makes a perfect lunch.

Serves: 4 to 6

1 pound organic ground beef
3 tablespoons taco seasoning
4 cups leafy greens
2 cups chopped mixed heirloom
   cherry tomatoes
3 avocados, halved, pitted, and diced

1. In a skillet or sauté pan over medium heat, sauté the beef for 3 to 5 minutes until browned. Stir in the taco seasoning. Cook until the beef is completely done and no longer pink.

2. Place the leafy greens in serving bowls.

3. Layer the beef over the greens.

4. Top each salad with tomatoes and avocado, and serve.

> **VARIATION TIP:** Top each salad with a dollop of full-fat coconut cream.

Shrimp, Bacon & Avocado Salad

Prep time: 5 minutes / **Cook time:** 10 minutes / **Total time:** 15 minutes

Shrimp and bacon go together like two peas in a pod. Okay, well not traditionally, but this salad is delicious and full of protein. Use deveined shrimp here as veined shrimp has tons of bacteria. Pick up deveined shrimp at a reliable seafood vendor. It's worth the extra cost so you don't have to spend a ton of time doing it yourself. This recipe also includes avocado, which adds a nice flavor, while the bacon gives this salad some crunch.

Serves: 4 to 6

1 (12-ounce) package
    nitrate-free bacon
1 pound peeled and deveined shrimp
1 cup freshly squeezed
    lemon juice, divided
2 avocados, halved, pitted, and sliced
2 large tomatoes, sliced
2 tablespoons EVOO
Sea salt
Freshly ground black pepper

1. In a skillet over medium heat, cook the bacon for about 5 minutes, or until cooked through. Transfer to paper towels to drain. Chop the bacon and set aside.

2. Wipe out the skillet and return it to medium heat. Add the shrimp. Cook for 4 to 5 minutes, stirring occasionally, until fully opaque. Add ½ cup of lemon juice.

3. Arrange the avocado slices on individual serving plates. Top each with the shrimp, bacon, and tomato slices.

4. In a small bowl, whisk the remaining ½ cup of lemon juice and the EVOO to combine. Season with sea salt and pepper. Pour the dressing over the salads or serve it on the side for everyone to help themselves.

> **VARIATION TIP:** Add 2 tablespoons of minced garlic to the skillet along with the shrimp.

Coconut Cream Fruit Salad

Prep time: 5 minutes / **Total time:** 5 minutes

This fruit salad will be the hit of your next party and will make you feel like a rock star. Choose the sweetest fruit you can find for this salad, even fruit that's verging on overripe. We top the salad with a drizzle of honey and fresh mint. It's the perfect fruit salad!

Serves: 4 to 6

4 cups mixed berries (such as sliced strawberries and blueberries)
3 cups cubed melon (cantaloupe, watermelon, honeydew, or a mix)
1 cup chopped fresh mint
2 tablespoons honey
2 tablespoons full-fat coconut cream

1. Grab a big serving bowl and toss together the berries and melon.

2. Gently mix the mint into the fruit.

3. Drizzle the fruit with the honey. Serve topped with coconut cream.

INGREDIENT TIP: Toss the fruit in freshly squeezed lemon juice to keep it from browning.

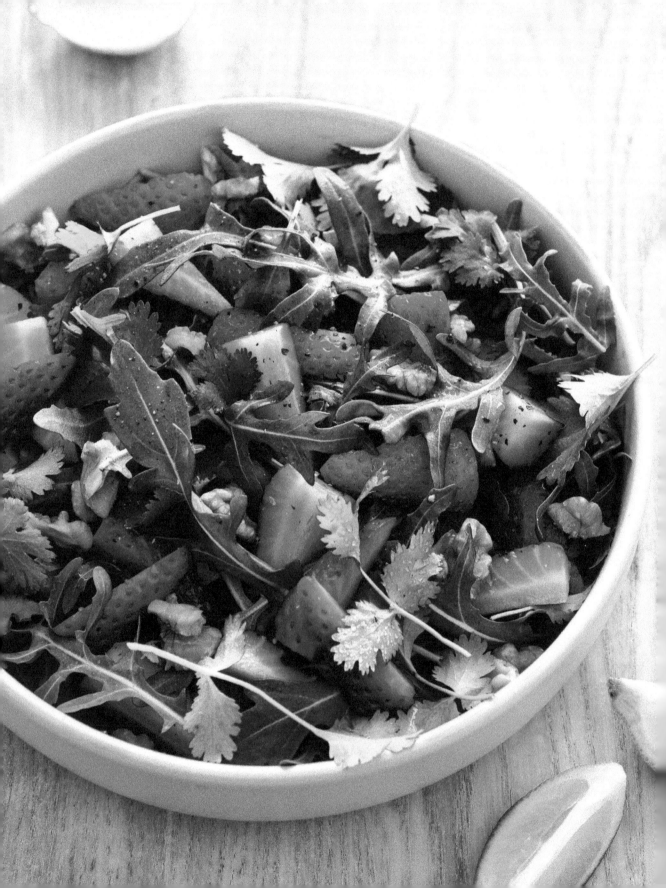

4

Easy Snacks, Appetizers & Sides

Oven-Fried Pickles 50

Strawberry & Arugula Side Salad 51

Mini Hamburgers 52

Bacon Jalapeño Poppers 53

Mini Pepperoni Pizza Bites 54

Marinara-Stuffed Mushrooms 55

Romaine Lettuce BLT Bites 56

Cauliflower Fried Rice 57

Sweet Potato Avocado Cups 58

Hearty Meatballs 59

Roasted Buffalo Cauliflower 60

Sweet Potato Fries 61

Avocado Oil Kale Chips 62

Salami-Wrapped Cantaloupe 63

Opposite: Strawberry & Arugula Side Salad, page 51

Oven-Fried Pickles

Prep time: 15 minutes / **Cook time:** 10 minutes / **Total time:** 25 minutes

These fried pickles are a crowd-pleasing appetizer. They also have far fewer calories than your traditional fried pickles because we use coconut flour instead of traditional flour.

Serves: 4 to 6

4 cups dill pickle chips
1 cup coconut flour
½ cup finely chopped fresh parsley
Sea salt
Freshly ground black pepper
1 cup full-fat coconut cream
1 large egg

1. Preheat the oven to 425°F. Line a baking sheet with parchment paper and set aside.

2. Drain the pickles and dry them with paper towels.

3. In a medium bowl, stir together the coconut flour and parsley. Season with sea salt and pepper.

4. In another medium bowl, whisk the coconut cream and the egg.

5. Take your time on this step so the breading sticks to each pickle: Dip each pickle in the coconut cream mixture, letting any excess fall back into the bowl, and into the flour mixture, making sure each is well coated. Place the coated pickle on the prepared baking sheet. Repeat with the remaining pickles.

6. Bake the pickles for 10 minutes, turning them halfway through the baking time, until lightly browned.

VARIATION TIP: Serve with Homemade Mayonnaise (page 126) for dipping.

Strawberry & Arugula Side Salad

Prep time: 5 minutes / Total time: 10 minutes

The combination of sweet strawberries and peppery arugula here will have your taste buds dancing. Pair it with Easy Barbecue Chicken (page 82), burgers, or pasta. It's flavorful, features ripe summer ingredients, and comes together in a jiffy! Use organic strawberries, as traditional strawberries are full of harmful chemicals (see The Dirty Dozen™, page 142, for more details). You can use either the lemon or lime juice version of Citrus Vinaigrette (page 134), but lime is my fave here.

Serves: 4 to 6

4 cups arugula
2 cups sliced fresh strawberries
1 cup chopped fresh cilantro
1 cup walnuts, toasted
Citrus Vinaigrette [page 134]

In a medium bowl, combine the arugula, strawberries, cilantro, and walnuts. Toss to combine. Drizzle the vinaigrette over the salad and serve.

SUBSTITUTION TIP: For a nut-free version, substitute sunflower or pumpkin seeds for the walnuts.

Mini Hamburgers

Prep time: 15 minutes / **Cook time:** 10 minutes / **Total time:** 25 minutes

These mini hamburgers are big on flavor and the cuteness factor, and they only take a few minutes to prep. Whip up a batch any time you need a fun snack for the kiddos or a hearty appetizer to pass at parties. These little burgers are also protein powerhouses with a whopping 60 grams of protein per burger!

Serves: 4 to 6

1½ pounds organic ground beef
½ medium red onion, chopped
Sea salt
Freshly ground black pepper
2 cups chopped iceberg lettuce
1 cup small pickle chips
2 cups cherry tomatoes, halved

1. In a medium bowl, mix together the ground beef and onion. Season with sea salt and pepper. Gently mix to combine. Shape the beef mixture into mini (1-inch) patties (18 to 20 patties).

2. Heat a grill pan or cast iron skillet over medium-high heat. When hot, place the patties in the pan. Cook for 2 to 3 minutes per side.

3. To assemble your mini burgers: Top a patty with some lettuce, a pickle, and a tomato half. Insert a toothpick into the mini burger to hold everything together. Repeat this step until you've made all your burgers.

> **VARIATION TIP:** Serve with Simple Ketchup (page 127) and Homemade Mayonnaise (on page 126).

Bacon Jalapeño Poppers

Prep time: 15 minutes / Cook time: 25 minutes / Total time: 40 minutes

If you love traditional jalapeño poppers, then this popping Paleo version is for you! These are packed with protein and work wonderfully for parties or as a weeknight appetizer. Save some of the coconut cream–chili powder filling to use as a dipping sauce.

Serves: 4 to 6

1 (12-ounce) can full-fat coconut cream
2 tablespoons chili powder
15 jalapeño peppers,
    halved and seeded
15 mini sausages (see tip)
15 nitrate-free bacon slices

1. Preheat the oven to 425°F. Line a baking sheet with parchment paper and set aside.

2. In a small bowl, stir together the coconut cream and chili powder until combined.

3. Fill each jalapeño half with about 2 tablespoons of the coconut cream mixture. Reserve the remaining coconut cream mixture for serving.

4. Place a mini sausage on top of each filled jalapeño.

5. Wrap each popper with 1 bacon slice and use a toothpick to secure it, if needed. Place the wrapped jalapeños on the prepared baking sheet.

6. Bake the poppers for 20 to 25 minutes until the bacon is cooked thoroughly.

INGREDIENT TIP: Use nitrate-free bacon and sausages; Applegate makes a great nitrate-free mini sausage.

Mini Pepperoni Pizza Bites

Prep time: 10 minutes / **Cook time:** 15 minutes / **Total time:** 25 minutes

Missing pepperoni pizza on the Paleo diet? Miss no more. These mini pepperoni pizza bites are for you! And the best part? They are loaded with veggies, so you not only get your recommended protein serving, but you also get your veggie serving with these nutrition-packed beasts. They make a great appetizer option when (surprise!) family comes for a visit or the neighbors pop in with their kiddos.

Serves: 4 to 6

12 slices nitrate-free pepperoni
(Applegate brand is very good)
2 cups chopped mixed bell peppers
1 (4-ounce) can sliced black olives
12 whole cherry tomatoes
2 cups Paleo Tomato Sauce (page 133)

1. Preheat the oven to 400°F.

2. Press 1 pepperoni slice into each well of a 12-cup muffin tin.

3. Fill each well with bell peppers, olives, and a cherry tomato.

4. Drizzle each pizza bite with about 2 tablespoons of Paleo Tomato Sauce.

5. Bake for 12 to 14 minutes, or until the sauce is bubbling and the pepperoni is nice and crispy.

> **VARIATION TIP:** Garnish with thinly sliced fresh basil leaves for extra flavor and because it makes them look pretty.

Marinara-Stuffed Mushrooms

Prep time: 10 minutes / **Cook time:** 10 minutes / **Total time:** 20 minutes

Stuffed mushrooms are usually loaded with cheese. Skip the cheese, save the fat, and use marinara sauce like I do. This recipe is also great if you have mushrooms you need to use up fast. With minimal ingredients, but tons of flavor these stuffed mushrooms will be a hit at your next party.

Serves: 4 to 6

1 (12-ounce) package cremini
   mushrooms, stemmed
¼ cup EVOO
Sea salt
Freshly ground black pepper
1 tablespoon garlic powder
2 cups marinara sauce
½ cup chopped fresh parsley
½ cup chopped fresh basil

1. Brush the mushrooms with EVOO and season with the sea salt, pepper, and garlic powder.

2. In a large skillet over medium heat, heat the remaining EVOO.

3. Place the mushrooms in the skillet. Cook for 5 minutes per side, or until tender. Transfer the mushrooms to a glass baking dish, hollow-side up.

4. Carefully fill each mushroom with marinara sauce.

5. Top with the parsley and basil.

6. If you like them crispy, place the mushrooms in a preheated 350°F oven for 5 minutes.

VARIATION TIP: For a meaty version of this dish, add crumbled cooked sausage (¼ to ½ pound) to the mushrooms before adding the sauce.

Romaine Lettuce BLT Bites

Prep time: 10 minutes / **Cook time:** 5 minutes / **Total time:** 15 minutes

BLT sammies are a favorite at my house for their amazing flavors, and I can easily make them anytime I want because I usually have the ingredients on hand. In fact, I always buy bacon in two-packs because we go through it so fast. That's what makes this recipe so great following the Paleo diet. You will get your BLT fix but without all the bread. These work as a fantastic side dish to eggs, bacon burgers, chicken—you name it. I use romaine lettuce; if you prefer iceberg lettuce, use it instead.

Serves: 4 to 6

1 (12-ounce) package
   nitrate-free bacon
2 cups sliced mixed tricolor
   cherry tomatoes
6 scallions, white and light
   green parts minced
¼ cup EVOO
1 cup freshly squeezed lemon juice
Sea salt
Freshly ground black pepper
1 head romaine lettuce,
   leaves separated

1. In a skillet over medium-high heat, cook the bacon for about 5 minutes until crispy. Transfer to paper towels to drain. Chop the bacon into small pieces.

2. In a medium bowl, combine the tomatoes, scallions, EVOO, and lemon juice. Season with sea salt and pepper. Gently stir to combine.

3. Fill each romaine lettuce leaf with some of the tomato mixture.

4. Sprinkle each stuffed romaine leaf with bacon and serve.

> **VARIATION TIP:** Garnish these bites with thinly sliced fresh basil.

Cauliflower Fried Rice

Prep time: 20 minutes / Cook time: 20 minutes / Total time: 40 minutes

You won't miss conventional fried rice once you try this cauliflower fried rice. The texture is the same and, with such vibrant flavors, this makes an unexpectedly delightful meal.

Serves: 4 to 6

2 tablespoons coconut oil, divided
1 pound boneless skinless chicken breast, thinly sliced
1 head cauliflower, cut into florets
1 tablespoon finely chopped peeled fresh ginger
3 large eggs, beaten
¼ cup coconut aminos

1. In a skillet over medium-high heat, heat 1 tablespoon of coconut oil.

2. Add the chicken. Cook for about 5 minutes until cooked through. Remove from the heat and set aside.

3. In a food processor, pulse the cauliflower until it resembles rice. Set aside.

4. Heat a large wok or skillet over medium-high heat and add the remaining 1 tablespoon of coconut oil.

5. Add the ginger and sauté until fragrant, about 1 minute.

6. Add the cooked chicken to the wok. Sauté for 3 minutes until heated through.

7. Add the cauliflower rice. Sauté for about 5 minutes until just tender.

8. Add the beaten eggs, scrambling them into the cauliflower.

9. Stir in the coconut aminos. Sauté everything for 5 minutes until browned.

VARIATION TIP: Add 1 cup of shredded carrots and 4 thinly sliced scallions after adding the ginger. Sauté for a few minutes until the carrots begin to soften. Garnish with ½ cup of chopped fresh cilantro.

Sweet Potato Avocado Cups

Prep time: 15 minutes / **Cook time:** 1 hour / **Total time:** 1 hour 15 minutes

Have a hankering for some carbs? Have no fear, because these sweet potato avocado cups will have you swooning. These cups make a great side dish or an unexpected appetizer. They have amazing flavor, are full of fiber, and are extremely filling. Top each sweet potato cup with additional coconut cream, if desired.

Serves: 4 to 6

4 sweet potatoes
1 tablespoon coconut oil, plus more, warmed, for serving (optional)
4 garlic cloves, peeled
1 avocado, halved, pitted, and sliced
1 cup chopped tomato
½ cup chopped red onion
1 cup chopped fresh cilantro
Sea salt
Freshly ground black pepper

1. Preheat the oven to 400°F.

2. Rub each sweet potato with a bit of the coconut oil and place on a baking sheet. Wrap the garlic cloves in a piece of aluminum foil and add to the baking sheet.

3. Bake the sweet potatoes and garlic for 1 hour, or until soft. When the potatoes are ready, their skins will peel off easily. Remove and let cool.

4. While the potatoes cool, in a food processor, combine the avocado, tomato, red onion, cilantro, and the roasted garlic cloves (popped from their skins). Pulse for 1 minute.

5. Slice the cooled sweet potatoes down the middle and scoop the avocado mixture into each sweet potato.

6. Season with sea salt and pepper. Drizzle with additional warmed coconut oil, if desired.

MAKE IT EASIER TIP: Instead of baking the sweet potatoes in the oven, cook them in the microwave (place on a microwave-safe plate, poke a few holes in them, and heat on high power for 5 to 10 minutes, until tender). You can also "roast" the garlic in the microwave. Cut the top off a whole, unpeeled head of garlic and place the head in a microwave-safe dish with a bit of water and a drizzle of olive oil. Cover and cook on high power in 2-minute intervals until the garlic is very soft. Squeeze the cooked cloves out of their skins to use.

Hearty Meatballs

Prep time: 15 minutes / Cook time: 40 minutes / Total time: 55 minutes

I think I've seen meatballs at every single party I've ever attended. Meatballs make a wonderful appetizer because they are easy to prepare, packed with protein, and flavorful when made correctly. My meatball recipe is especially delicious because the fresh herbs make the flavors burst. I include red onion for a bit of a zesty flavor. Make these for your family tonight and I bet they will be added to your weekly dinner rotation (you may want to double the recipe to serve this as a main dish).

Serves: 4 to 6

1 pound organic ground beef
1 large egg, beaten
1 medium red onion, minced
2 garlic cloves, minced
¼ cup minced fresh parsley, plus additional for garnishing

1. Preheat the oven to 400°F. Line a rimmed baking sheet with parchment paper and set aside.

2. In a large bowl, combine the beef, egg, red onion, garlic, and parsley. Mix, making sure to really knead the ingredients together to get the meatball mixture nice and thick. Form the meat mixture into 1-inch balls and place them on the prepared baking sheet.

3. Bake the meatballs for 40 minutes, or until cooked through and no longer pink.

4. Serve the meatballs hot, garnished with parsley.

VARIATION TIP: Serve with Simple Ketchup [page 127] and Homemade Mayonnaise [page 126] for dipping.

Roasted Buffalo Cauliflower

Prep time: 15 minutes / **Cook time:** 15 minutes / **Total time:** 30 minutes

This recipe will remind you of Buffalo wings, and it pairs well with the Bacon-Wrapped Chicken Wings (page 84). These make a great appetizer, although they do fall on the semi-hot side so be sure the kiddos like the heat before offering them any. Serve these spicy bites with Paleo Ranch Dressing (page 137) and spice up your next football party.

Serves: 4 to 6

1 head cauliflower, cut into florets
3 teaspoons paprika
3 teaspoons garlic powder
2 teaspoons ground cumin
Sea salt
Freshly ground black pepper
1 cup freshly squeezed lemon juice
½ cup hot sauce (Tessemae's is a
    great Paleo-friendly brand)
2 tablespoons ghee, melted

1. Preheat the oven to 425°F. Line a rimmed baking sheet with parchment paper and set aside.

2. Place the cauliflower in a large bowl and set aside.

3. In a small bowl, stir together the paprika, garlic powder, and cumin. Season with sea salt and pepper, and stir again to combine.

4. In another small bowl, stir together the lemon juice, hot sauce, and melted ghee. Spread the mixture over the florets.

5. Coat each floret in the spice mixture. Spread the florets evenly on the prepared baking sheet.

6. Bake for 10 to 15 minutes, or until the florets are crispy.

> SUBSTITUTION TIP: To make this recipe vegan, substitute coconut oil or olive oil for the ghee.

Sweet Potato Fries

Prep time: 20 minutes / **Cook time:** 30 minutes / **Total time:** 50 minutes

Sweet potato fries pair nicely with a big, juicy protein burger. One cup of sweet potatoes gives you more than the recommended daily allowance of vitamin A, which is a form of beta-carotene. Beta-carotene is essential for eye, skin, and heart health—our bodies need it. And vitamin A is especially important for women of reproductive age. Vitamin A is essential to a healthy menstrual cycle. Eating sweet potatoes does a body good!

Serves: 4 to 6

2 pounds sweet potatoes, skin
   on, cut into large wedges
¼ cup EVOO
¼ cup coconut oil
¼ cup minced fresh rosemary leaves
1 tablespoon flaky sea salt
Paleo Ranch Dressing (page 137),
   for serving

1. Preheat the oven to 425°F. Line a baking sheet with parchment paper and set aside.

2. In a large bowl, combine the sweet potato wedges, EVOO, and coconut oil. Mix with clean hands to coat the sweet potatoes in the oil. Place the sweet potatoes on the prepared baking sheet, spreading them in a single layer so they cook evenly.

3. Roast for 20 to 30 minutes, or until they reach a nice golden brown.

4. Top with the rosemary and sea salt, and serve with the Paleo Ranch Dressing for dipping.

> SUBSTITUTION TIP: To make this recipe vegan, skip the dressing.

Avocado Oil Kale Chips

Prep time: 10 minutes / Cook time: 25 minutes / Total time: 35 minutes

Kale chips make tasty use of leftover kale that needs to be used up fast. This recipe can also help feed that salty craving that gets us from time to time. These chips are crunchy and filled with healthy fats from the avocado oil, which makes them even better for you! Plus, why spend your hard-earned money on chips at the grocery store when you can make them yourself?

Serves: 4 to 6

2 teaspoons paprika
2 teaspoons onion powder
1 teaspoon garlic powder
Zest of 1 lemon
1 to 2 bunches green leaf
   kale, thoroughly washed
   and dried, stemmed
2 to 4 tablespoons avocado oil
Chunky sea salt [chunky sea
   salt is flakier salt that works
   well as a topping]

1. Preheat the oven to 350°F.

2. In a small bowl, stir together the paprika, onion powder, garlic powder, and lemon zest.

3. Cut the kale leaves into smaller sizes, about the size of a potato chip. Place the kale in a large bowl and drizzle with the avocado oil. Massage the oil into the leaves to make sure they are all well coated.

4. Sprinkle the spice blend over the kale. Use clean hands to combine everything thoroughly. Spread the kale in a single layer on a baking sheet (or use two baking sheets if necessary).

5. Bake for 10 minutes. Rotate the baking sheet(s) from back to front and top to bottom if using more than one sheet. Bake for 15 minutes more, or until the chips are nice and crispy.

6. Sprinkle with chunky sea salt!

PRO TIP: For the crunchiest chips, dry your kale leaves very well, tear them into large pieces, and use dry spices and only a bit of oil, as liquid flavorings will prevent your chips from crisping up.

Salami-Wrapped Cantaloupe

Prep time: 10 minutes / Total time: 10 minutes

Salami is delicious with anything, but have you tried it with fruit? If you haven't, you need to make this recipe right now because it will knock your socks off. This is the easiest snack ever and all you need besides the ingredients are toothpicks. No cooking involved.

Serves: 4 to 6

12 ounces nitrate-free salami slices
1 cantaloupe, sliced, seeded, and cubed (you could also use a melon baller)
½ cup balsamic vinegar
⅓ cup EVOO
½ cup chopped fresh mint
Flaky sea salt
Freshly ground black pepper

1. Wrap a slice of salami around each piece of cantaloupe, securing it with a toothpick. Repeat until all the melon is wrapped in salami. Place the wrapped melon on a plate.

2. Drizzle with the vinegar and EVOO.

3. Garnish with mint and season with flaky sea salt and pepper.

VARIATION TIP: Fancy this snack up by using prosciutto instead of salami.

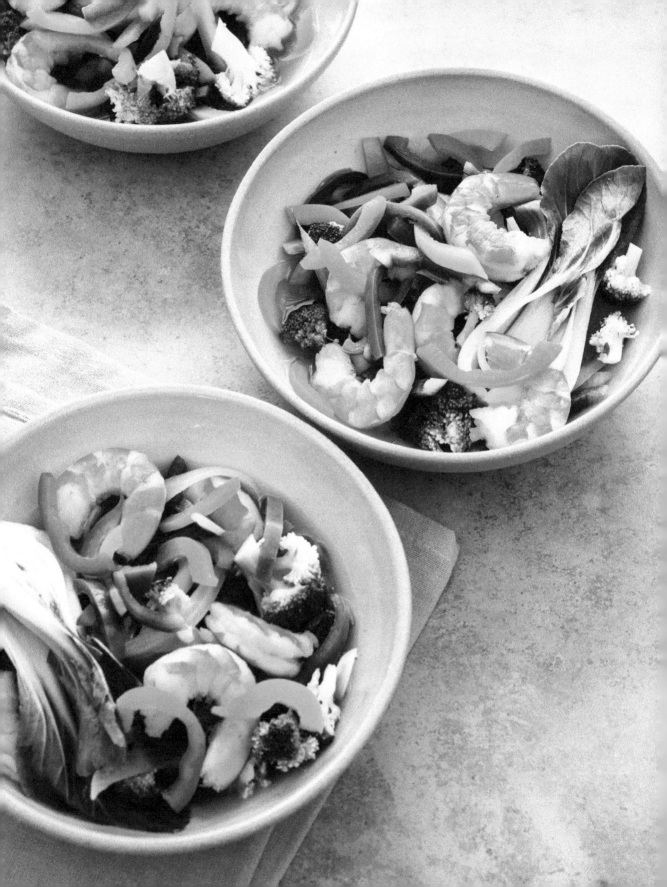

5

Fish & Seafood Mains

Opposite: Bok Choy Shrimp Soup, page 71

Lemon & Roasted Garlic Tilapia

Prep time: 5 minutes / **Cook time:** 15 minutes / **Total time:** 20 minutes

Tilapia is a wonderful fish because it's affordable, light, and easy to make. There is no real way to mess up tilapia as long as you have some oil, lemon, fresh garlic, and an oven. It's a perfect starter fish for those who are either new to fish or don't eat it a lot.

Serves: 4 to 6

4 to 6 (6-ounce) tilapia fillets
2 tablespoons EVOO
1 lemon, halved
Sea salt
Freshly ground black pepper
6 garlic cloves, roasted and
    peeled (see tip)
½ cup finely chopped fresh parsley

1. Preheat the oven to 350°F. Line a baking sheet with parchment paper.

2. Place the tilapia fillets on the prepared baking sheet and brush them with the EVOO.

3. Slice one lemon half into rounds. Squeeze the juice from the other half over the fish.

4. Sprinkle the fish with sea salt and pepper.

5. Place the roasted garlic cloves around the fish. Top the fish with the lemon slices.

6. Roast for 15 minutes, or until the tilapia is nice and crispy. Garnish with fresh parsley and serve.

> PRO TIP: To roast garlic, slice the top off a whole head of garlic exposing the cloves, drizzle it with EVOO, and wrap in aluminum foil. Roast in a 400°F oven for about 1 hour. Squeeze the roasted garlic cloves out of their skins to use.

Lemon-Dill Salmon

Prep time: 15 minutes / Cook time: 20 minutes / Total time: 35 minutes

If you are a fish lover, you will love this easy salmon dish, which pairs nicely with cauliflower rice. When purchasing salmon, always choose fresh wild-caught salmon. The higher the grade the better it is. It's a bit pricier but worth the extra money. Opt for king or Chinook; a less expensive, but still wonderful, option is sockeye.

Serves: 4 to 6

For the lemon-dill sauce

⅓ cup Homemade Mayonnaise (page 126), or store-bought mayo
Juice of 1 lemon
½ cup finely chopped fresh dill, a few sprigs reserved for the fish
1 garlic clove, minced

For the salmon

4 to 6 (6-ounce) salmon fillets
2 tablespoons EVOO
2 lemons, divided
Sea salt
Freshly ground black pepper

Preheat the oven to 375°F.

To make the lemon-dill sauce

1. In a medium bowl, stir together the mayonnaise and lemon juice.

2. Add the chopped dill and garlic to the mayonnaise. Stir to combine. Cover and stash in the fridge until ready to use.

To make the salmon

1. Place the salmon fillets in a baking dish and drizzle with EVOO and the juice of 1 lemon. Season with sea salt and pepper.

2. Spoon dill sauce over each fillet. Slice the remaining lemon into 4 to 6 rounds and top each fillet with 1 lemon slice.

3. Place the reserved dill sprigs around the fillets in the baking dish for extra flavor.

4. Bake for 20 minutes, or until the fish flakes easily with a fork.

> VARIATION TIP: Add 2 sliced scallions and 1 to 2 tablespoons of capers to the dill sauce for extra flavor.

Shrimp Kabobs

Prep time: 10 minutes / Cook time: 15 minutes / Total time: 25 minutes

I love kabobs. They are easy to make and do not take a ton of thought. They are especially great if you have access to a grill; if not, make these in the oven on a baking sheet. Shrimp is one of my favorite seafoods because it's flavorful and light. Shrimp is awesome for its high protein content and it's relatively inexpensive to purchase. I love adding bell peppers to kabobs but use any veggies you like—make it a crunchy veggie though. Don't go crazy with too many veggies or you will take away from the flavor of the shrimp. I've added mango to these skewers, but you can add a fruit of your choice. Pineapple is good, too.

Serves: 4 to 6

1½ pounds shrimp, peeled and deveined
1 lemon, sliced
1 head garlic, cloves separated and peeled
1 mango, peeled and cubed
Tricolor bell peppers, as many as you like, cored and cut into squares
2 tablespoons ghee, melted

1. Preheat a grill to its hottest setting.

2. Grab some skewers (8 to 10) and place a shrimp on each.

3. Add a lemon slice and a whole garlic clove to each.

4. Add a cube of mango and a square of bell pepper. Repeat until the skewers are full and all the ingredients are used.

5. Brush the skewers with melted ghee.

6. Place your skewers on the grill. Cook for 10 to 12 minutes, or until the veggies and fruit are tender and the shrimp is pink and cooked through.

PREPARATION TIP: If you don't have access to an outdoor grill, make these on the stovetop in a grill pan set over high heat. Alternatively, arrange the skewers in a baking dish and roast them in a preheated 400°F oven for about 15 minutes.

Tuna Salad Cups

Prep time: 5 minutes / Total time: 5 minutes

Tuna salad cups are a fantastic quick meal option. All you need are a few key ingredients and this meal literally takes 5 minutes to make. It's refreshing made with iceberg lettuce, which is cool and crunchy. You can whip these up so fast and have them ready in time for friends coming over or for when the kiddos get home from school and need a healthy snack. Make this for dinner tonight and pair it with a refreshing glass of white wine. And just like that, dinner is served!

Serves: 4 to 6

2 cups cooked tuna, flaked

2 cups minced celery

6 scallions, white and light green parts chopped, 2 tablespoons reserved for garnishing

Homemade Mayonnaise (page 126)

Sea salt

1 head iceberg lettuce, leaves separated

1. In a medium bowl, stir together the tuna, celery, scallions, and mayonnaise. Season with sea salt to taste.

2. Place as many lettuce leaves as you like on small plates or in shallow serving bowls.

3. Top each with a scoop of tuna salad. Serve garnished with the reserved scallions.

VARIATION TIP: Add 1 cup of halved cherry tomatoes and ½ cup of chopped fresh cilantro to the mix for additional flavor.

Sushi Bowls

Prep time: 10 minutes / **Total time:** 10 minutes

Sushi is awesome, but it's typically wrapped in rice no matter the restaurant serving it. My Paleo sushi bowl has lots of protein from fresh tuna and you get your vitamin fix from the seaweed. The avocado gives this bowl a healthy fat boost. You also get an inflammation fighter with the fresh ginger. Seaweed is so good for you—but it is not used enough in the standard American diet. This bowl will fulfill your recommended daily allowance of vitamins.

Serves: 4 to 6

1 pound fresh tuna, thinly sliced

1 avocado, halved, pitted, and sliced

1 Japanese cucumber, thinly sliced

1 (1-ounce) package dried seaweed
sheets, cut into strips

1 cup coconut aminos

2 tablespoons minced peeled
fresh ginger (optional)

1. Divide the tuna, avocado, cucumber, and seaweed sheets evenly among 4 to 6 serving bowls.

2. Drizzle with the coconut aminos. Top with the ginger (if using).

VARIATION TIP: Garnish with 2 tablespoons of toasted sesame seeds for added flavor, texture, and a boost of antioxidants.

Bok Choy Shrimp Soup

Prep time: 10 minutes / Cook time: 20 minutes / Total time: 30 minutes

Bok choy is a delicious vegetable that is a nutritious powerhouse. It's full of fiber and B vitamins and is great for detoxifying your system, keeping your skin clear, and helping to keep "things" moving. Eat this powerful little veggie as much as you like because it's really good for you. The other star of the show here is broccoli, one of my favorite veggies. It has actually been shown to reduce cancer risk and is wonderful for managing menstrual cycles. It's a vegetable that everyone should eat more often. This soup is fun to make and is a feast for the eyes as well as the tummy.

Serves: 4 to 6

1½ pounds shrimp, peeled and deveined

2 tablespoons minced peeled fresh ginger, plus more for garnishing (optional)

3 garlic cloves, minced, plus more for garnishing (optional)

4 cups organic chicken stock

1½ pounds bok choy, trimmed

1. In a medium saucepan over medium high heat, combine the shrimp, ginger, garlic, and chicken stock. Bring to a simmer. Cook for 3 to 5 minutes until the shrimp is cooked through.

2. Add the bok choy. Cook for 5 to 10 minutes more until the bok choy is crisp-tender.

3. Serve the soup garnished with more garlic and ginger, if desired.

> VARIATION TIP: Make this as a stir-fry rather than a soup. Leave out the chicken stock and instead heat 2 tablespoons coconut oil in a large skillet over medium heat. Add the ginger and garlic. Cook for about 3 minutes until softened. Add the bok choy. Cook for about 5 minutes, stirring, until it begins to soften. Add the shrimp. Cook for 3 to 5 minutes more until the shrimp is cooked through and the bok choy is crisp-tender.

Lobster & Mango Salad

Prep time: 10 minutes / **Total time:** 10 minutes

I find lobster to be one of those foods you either love or hate. It has a pretty interesting flavor and texture. If you enjoy lobster, you'll love this lobster and mango salad. This recipe also includes hard-boiled eggs, which pair nicely with the lobster. You may think that mango and eggs are a strange flavor combination, but they actually complement each other really well. This is a basic, healthy, refreshing salad that can be served for dinner or lunch.

Serves: 4 to 6

6 cups arugula, rinsed
2 mangos, peeled and diced
6 large hard-boiled eggs, sliced
1 garlic clove, minced
1 pound cooked lobster meat, chopped
Dressing of choice [see
    chapter 9], for serving

1. In a medium serving bowl, combine the arugula, mango, eggs, and garlic.

2. Top the salad with the cooked lobster meat and serve. Pass the dressing on the side.

> **VARIATION TIP:** Add ½ cup of chopped fresh parsley to the salad for added color and flavor.

Fish Tacos

Prep time: 10 minutes / Total time: 15 minutes

If you love fish and you love tacos then you are going to love my fish taco recipe, made with light, delicious tilapia. This recipe calls for Cauliflower Tortillas (page 139); prepare the tortillas before you dive into this recipe. These fish tacos are easy and healthy, and are a great dinner any night of the week!

Serves: 4 to 6

1 recipe Cauliflower Tortillas
   (page 139), for serving
2 pounds tilapia, cooked and sliced
1 cup diced Roma tomatoes
1 medium red onion, diced
½ cup chopped fresh cilantro

Fill the tortillas with the tilapia, tomatoes, red onion, and cilantro. Serve immediately.

VARIATION TIP: To add a whole lot of color and flavor, garnish these tacos with thinly sliced purple cabbage, salsa, and a squeeze of fresh lime juice.

Bacon-Wrapped Shrimp

Prep time: 15 minutes / Cook time: 25 minutes / Total time: 40 minutes

Bacon and shrimp are a perfect match. The richness of the bacon complements the shrimp and gives this dish 12 grams of protein per serving, which is a good amount for a meal, especially on the Paleo diet. You may be concerned about sodium in this recipe, but as long as you opt for nitrate-free bacon, you will be fine. The zesty lemon juice and fresh cilantro give the dish a zing. Devein your shrimp before cooking.

Serves: 4 to 6

½ cup freshly squeezed lemon juice
¼ cup EVOO
½ cup chopped fresh cilantro
1 garlic clove, minced
1 pound shrimp, peeled and deveined
1 (12-ounce) package nitrate-free
 bacon, strips halved widthwise

1. Preheat the oven to 350°F. Line a baking sheet with parchment paper and set aside.

2. In a large bowl, whisk the lemon juice, EVOO, cilantro, and garlic.

3. Add the shrimp to the dressing. Gently mix to coat the shrimp evenly.

4. Wrap each shrimp in a piece of bacon and place on the prepared baking sheet.

5. Bake for 20 to 25 minutes until the bacon is nice and crispy.

VARIATION TIP: Serve these with hot sauce or Paleo Ranch Dressing (page 137) for dipping.

Parsley & Garlic Scallops

Prep time: 10 minutes / Cook time: 10 minutes / Total time: 20 minutes

Scallops are classic. They pair well with red wine and are delicious drenched in garlic. If you've never cooked scallops at home, not to worry; they are easy to cook in the comfort of your own kitchen. Purchase the freshest scallops you can find from a high-quality seafood vendor or a local farmers' market and cook them the same day. Seafood doesn't do well sitting in the fridge.

Serves: 4 to 6

⅓ cup EVOO
4 garlic cloves, minced
1½ pounds sea scallops
1 tablespoon paprika
Juice of 2 lemons, plus zest from the lemons reserved for garnishing
½ cup minced fresh parsley, 2 tablespoons reserved for garnishing
Sea salt
Freshly ground black pepper

1. In a large skillet over medium heat, heat the EVOO. Add the garlic and stir.

2. Add the scallops to the skillet and season with the paprika.

3. Add the lemon juice and parsley. Cook the scallops for 2 to 3 minutes per side to sear.

4. Serve the scallops warm, seasoned with sea salt and pepper, and garnished with the reserved lemon zest and parsley.

VARIATION TIP: Bacon is a flavorful counterpart to delicately flavored scallops. Take this dish up a notch: Add 2 or 3 bacon slices, chopped, to the skillet along with the garlic. Cook for a few minutes until the bacon begins to brown before adding the scallops.

Salmon Burgers

Prep time: 5 minutes / Cook time: 20 minutes / Total time: 25 minutes

Salmon burgers may sound complicated to make, but are actually a lot easier than you might think. All you need for these delicious burgers is what you would normally need for regular burgers with a few ingredients swapped out.

Serves: 4 to 6

1½ pounds salmon
2 large eggs
1 red onion, chopped
½ cup minced fresh dill
1 teaspoon red pepper flakes (optional)
Sea salt
Freshly ground black pepper
1 tablespoon EVOO
4 to 6 cooked sweet potatoes, cooled, peeled, and halved through the middle lengthwise (for buns)
Sliced pickles, for serving (optional)

1. In a large bowl, combine the salmon, eggs, red onion, dill, and red pepper flakes (if using). Gently stir to combine. Season with sea salt and black pepper. Form the mixture into 4 to 6 patties.

2. In a large skillet over medium-high heat, heat the EVOO.

3. Add the salmon patties (you may have to work in batches). Cook for about 5 minutes per side until nicely browned and crisp on the outside and cooked through.

4. Serve on a sweet potato "bun" with a pickle slice (if using) and other toppings as desired.

VARIATION TIP: Serve with Homemade Mayonnaise (page 126) or Paleo Ranch Dressing (page 137).

Salmon & Peaches

Prep time: 5 minutes / Cook time: 25 minutes / Total time: 30 minutes

I call this recipe good mood food. Salmon is chock-full of omega-3s, which our bodies need to function properly. Most of us don't get enough in our food. This recipe also has peaches, which are among my favorite fruits and are even tastier when roasted. The combination of foods in this recipe gives your body the fuel it needs and delivers it in tasty fashion!

Serves: 4 to 6

½ cup EVOO, plus more for drizzling
½ cup finely chopped fresh cilantro
1 medium red onion, diced
2 tablespoons minced
   peeled fresh ginger
Sea salt
Freshly ground black pepper
4 to 6 (6-ounce) salmon fillets
4 cups sliced fresh peaches

1. Preheat the oven to 350°F. Line a baking sheet with parchment paper and set aside.

2. In a small bowl, whisk the EVOO, cilantro, red onion, and ginger. Season with sea salt and pepper. Whisk again to combine.

3. Place the salmon on the baking sheet and brush the cilantro dressing over it, giving it a nice coat.

4. Place the sliced peaches on top of and around the salmon. Drizzle the peaches with EVOO.

5. Bake the salmon and peaches for 20 to 25 minutes, or until the salmon is nice and crispy and the peaches are nicely browned.

> VARIATION TIP: Use sliced fresh pineapple rings instead of the peaches for a more tropical flavor.

Lemon-Garlic Shrimp & Tomatoes

Prep time: 5 minutes / **Cook time:** 15 minutes / **Total time:** 20 minutes

Lemon, garlic, and shrimp go together so well, which is why you'll see this recipe in so many fancy restaurants. But, no need to spend $100 and leave the house to get a delicious meal like this. Simply pick up some shrimp on your way home and watch Netflix on the couch. Instead of using butter in this recipe, as is traditional, I use ghee. Grab some fresh lemons and some cherry tomatoes and let's get cooking!

Serves: 4 to 6

½ cup ghee
1½ pounds shrimp, peeled
    and deveined
6 to 8 garlic cloves, minced
1 cup chopped fresh basil,
    2 tablespoons reserved
    for garnishing
1 cup chopped fresh cilantro,
    2 tablespoons reserved
    for garnishing
2 cups heirloom cherry tomatoes
2 lemons, halved

1. In a sauté pan or large skillet over medium-high heat, heat the ghee. Add the shrimp. Cook for 2 to 5 minutes until it starts to turn pink.

2. Sprinkle the minced garlic over the shrimp. Add the basil and cilantro, and toss to combine. Sauté everything for a few minutes more until the shrimp is mostly cooked.

3. Add the cherry tomatoes. Sauté for 5 minutes more until the tomatoes start to pop. Transfer to serving dishes. Squeeze fresh lemon juice over everything. Garnish with the reserved basil and cilantro.

> MAKE IT EASIER TIP: Buy shrimp that has already been peeled and deveined. It costs a bit more, but will save you a ton of prep time.

Coconut-Crusted Calamari

Prep time: 10 minutes / Cook time: 10 minutes / Total time: 20 minutes

Think you can't have calamari on the Paleo diet? Think again. This is a really easy recipe. It's healthier than traditional calamari and has less fat. Although this recipe does use coconut oil to fry the calamari, it's lower in fat than other oils and burns at a higher heat so the calamari will be done faster. Keep your eye on the calamari so you do not overcook it! You have to work quickly so read the recipe through before starting.

Serves: 4 to 6

1 cup ghee, melted
2 cups unsweetened
   shredded coconut
2 cups coconut flour
4 cups coconut oil
1⅓ pounds cleaned squid, cut into rings
Flaky sea salt
¼ cup freshly squeezed lemon juice
Cocktail sauce, for serving

1. Place the melted ghee in a medium bowl. In another medium bowl, whisk the coconut and coconut flour.

2. In a deep skillet over medium heat, melt the coconut oil, letting it get really hot. You'll know when the oil is ready when it begins to bubble slightly.

3. Dip a piece of calamari into the ghee and dip it into the coconut mixture, coating the calamari really well. Repeat to coat all the calamari.

4. Using a slotted spoon, carefully place several pieces of calamari into the hot oil, but be careful not to crowd the pan. Cook for 30 seconds to 1 minute until browned. Using a slotted spoon, transfer to paper towels to drain. Repeat until all the calamari is cooked.

5. Sprinkle the calamari with sea salt, drizzle with lemon juice, and serve with the cocktail sauce for dipping.

PRO TIP: To minimize mess when deep-frying, use a high-sided pot, such as a Dutch oven. A cast iron Dutch oven (either enameled or uncoated) makes a great deep-frying pot because it conducts heat well and contains splatters.

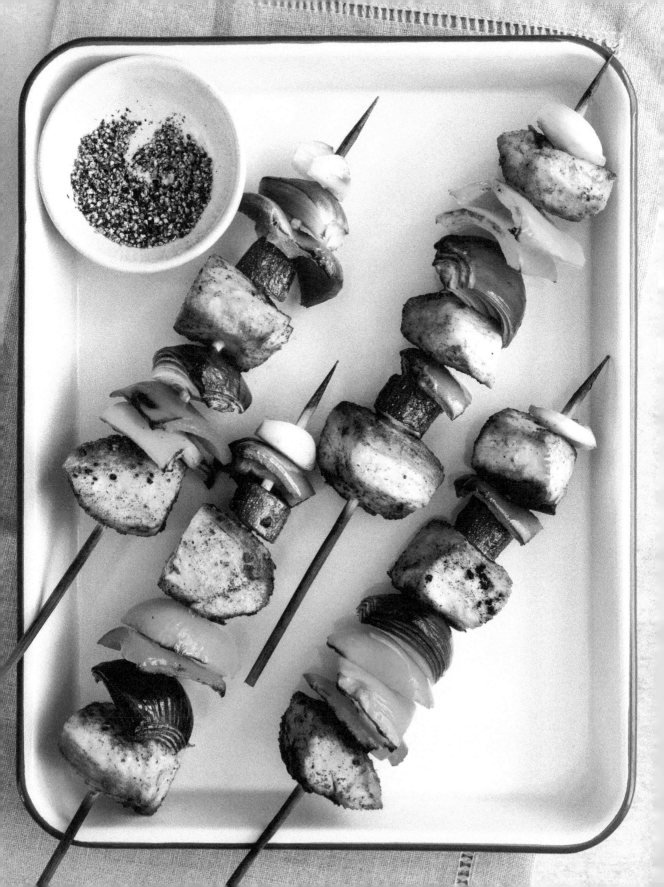

6

Poultry Mains

Opposite: Chicken & Veggie Shish Kabobs, page 85

Easy Barbecue Chicken

Prep time: 15 minutes / **Cook time:** 1 hour / **Total time:** 1 hour 15 minutes

Barbecued chicken equals summer fun, but many people think they are not "allowed" to have it on the Paleo diet. Not true. As long as you make your own Barbecue Sauce (see page 132) or buy a sugar-free, chemical-free version, you can totally eat barbecue chicken on the Paleo diet. And this chicken is good—really good. It is oven-baked here, but grill it if you prefer.

Serves: 4 to 6

2 cups Barbecue Sauce (page 132) or store-bought sugar-free chemical-free barbecue sauce
3 tablespoons coconut aminos
1 teaspoon chili powder
Sea salt
Freshly ground black pepper
4 to 6 chicken legs

1. Preheat the oven to 425°F. Line a baking sheet with parchment paper and set aside.

2. In a small bowl, stir together the barbecue sauce, coconut aminos, and chili powder. Season with sea salt and pepper. Stir again to combine.

3. Using a pastry brush, coat each chicken leg with the sauce and then give each leg a second coat. Place the basted legs on the prepared baking sheet 1 inch apart.

4. Bake for 50 to 60 minutes until the chicken is nice and crispy and the juices run clear.

> **VARIATION TIP:** For smoky flavor, cook this chicken on the grill. Preheat a grill to medium-high heat. Coat the chicken in the sauce mixture and place it on the grill. Cook for 20 to 30 minutes, basting occasionally with the remaining sauce mixture and turning halfway through cooking, until cooked through.

Veggie & Chicken Bake

Prep time: 10 minutes / Cook time: 50 minutes / Total time: 1 hour

Did your grandmother make chicken and rice casserole? Mine did, all the time when I was a child—and I LOVED it! There is something so cozy and comforting about a good chicken casserole. Well, if you enjoy chicken casserole as much as I do, you will love my amped-up veggie version. This chicken and veggie bake provides your fiber fill and an ample amount of protein.

Serves: 4 to 6

1 cup coconut aminos
1½ pounds boneless skinless
    chicken breast, cubed
2 tablespoons chopped garlic
Sea salt
Freshly ground black pepper
2 cups broccoli florets
2 cups sliced green beans
1 medium red onion, diced

1. Preheat the oven to 350°F.

2. Place the coconut aminos in a skillet and place the skillet over medium-high heat.

3. Add the chicken and garlic. Season with sea salt and pepper. Cook the chicken for 10 minutes, or until it's no longer pink in the middle.

4. Place half each of the broccoli, green beans, and red onion in a casserole dish in a single layer.

5. Add the chicken. Top the chicken with the remaining veggies.

6. Bake for 40 to 50 minutes until everything is nice and crispy.

> VARIATION TIP: Substitute other nonstarchy veggies you have on hand. Mushrooms, asparagus, bell peppers, and summer squash all work well here.

Bacon-Wrapped Chicken Wings

Prep time: 15 minutes / **Cook time:** 50 minutes / **Total time:** 1 hour 5 minutes

You can't have a Paleo cookbook and not include this recipe. Bacon-wrapped chicken is simple, good home cooking. I like to make this on Friday night just to enjoy the leftovers for lunch over the weekend.

Serves: 4 to 6

1 cup Barbecue Sauce (page 132)
2 teaspoons cayenne pepper
2 tablespoons chopped garlic
1½ pounds chicken wings
1 (12-ounce) package nitrate-free bacon, strips halved lengthwise

1. Preheat the oven to 400°F. Line a baking sheet with parchment paper and set aside.

2. In a medium bowl, stir together the barbecue sauce, cayenne, and garlic. Add the chicken wings and stir to coat each wing with barbecue sauce.

3. Wrap 1 bacon slice around each chicken wing and place on the prepared baking sheet. Continue with the remaining bacon and chicken until all are wrapped.

4. Bake for 40 to 50 minutes until the chicken is cooked and the bacon is nice and crispy.

> PRO TIP: For perfectly crispy wings, rinse the chicken wings and dry them thoroughly with paper towels before coating in the sauce.

Chicken & Veggie Shish Kabobs

Prep time: 15 minutes / Cook time: 25 minutes / Total time: 40 minutes

Made with a bunch of fresh veggies and a handful of pantry staples, this flavorful recipe is a summer classic and a great recipe for Memorial Day!

Serves: 4 to 6

2 tablespoons ghee
1 tablespoon ground cumin
1 tablespoon sea salt
2 teaspoons freshly ground
    black pepper
1½ pounds boneless skinless
    chicken breast, cubed
3 bell peppers, a mix of
    colors, stemmed, seeded,
    and cut into squares
1 zucchini, sliced into rounds
1 medium red onion, chopped
    into squares

1. In a skillet over medium-high heat, heat the ghee. Add the cumin, sea salt, and pepper.

2. Add the chicken to the skillet. Cook for 15 minutes, stirring occasionally, or until cooked thoroughly. Set aside.

3. Using 6 skewers, alternate placing bell pepper, zucchini, chicken, and red onion on them. Wrap the shish kabobs in aluminum foil.

4. Preheat a grill to medium-high heat or a cast iron skillet over medium-high heat.

5. Place the wrapped skewers on the grill (or skillet, if using). Cook for 5 to 10 minutes until the veggies are nice and crispy.

VARIATION TIP: Add fresh pineapple chunks to the skewers for a tropical flavor twist.

Chicken Coconut Cream Casserole

Prep time: 15 minutes / **Cook time:** 50 minutes / **Total time:** 1 hour 5 minutes

This creamy chicken casserole is rich and tastes like a coconut dream. Because it's dairy-free it also freezes well. Make this meal on a Sunday and have it ready to go for the entire week.

Serves: 4 to 6

Coconut oil spray, for preparing
   the baking dish
1 pound boneless skinless cooked
   chicken breast, cubed
2 cups full-fat coconut cream
2 cups chopped broccoli
2 cups chopped baby carrots
2 cups unsweetened
   shredded coconut

1. Preheat the oven to 350°F. Coat a casserole dish with coconut oil spray.

2. Place the chicken in the prepared dish in a single layer.

3. Spread half the coconut cream on top of the chicken.

4. Add a layer of half each of the broccoli and carrots.

5. Spread the remaining half of the coconut cream on top.

6. Finish with the remaining broccoli and carrots.

7. Top the casserole with the shredded coconut. Cover the casserole tightly with aluminum foil.

8. Bake for 50 minutes, or until crispy.

MAKE IT EASIER TIP: Use leftover roasted chicken or buy a rotisserie chicken from the supermarket (just be sure to check the ingredients!) to cut out a whole lot of prep time.

5-Ingredient Chili

Prep time: 15 minutes / Cook time: 8 hours / Total time: 8 hours 15 minutes

Chili is pure comfort food—and you can look forward to some comforting leftovers for the entire week. You can get really creative with those leftovers, too. Load them into a sweet potato or add the leftover chili to Cauliflower Tortillas (page 139) and make tacos. The possibilities are endlessly delicious.

Serves: 4 to 6

1½ pounds organic free-
 range ground chicken
2 cups chopped zucchini
1 cup sliced black olives
4 cups cauliflower rice
2 tablespoons chili powder
Sea salt
Freshly ground black pepper

1. In a skillet over medium heat, cook the ground chicken for 4 to 6 minutes until browned. You should not need any oil as the oil naturally comes from the meat. Transfer the cooked chicken to a slow cooker.

2. Add the zucchini, olives, cauliflower rice, and chili powder. Gently stir to combine everything.

3. Cover the cooker and set to high heat. Cook for 8 hours. The longer it cooks, the better it will taste. Serve hot.

> VARIATION TIP: This recipe is great for serving a crowd, and you can make it go even further by adding additional veggies such as cubed sweet potatoes, corn kernels, diced bell peppers, diced toma-toes, or sliced mushrooms.

Chicken Fajita Bowls

Prep time: 5 minutes / **Cook time:** 15 minutes / **Total time:** 20 minutes

Make these easy fajita bowls tonight and you will be so happy and satisfied. These bowls are filling and provide your protein and veggies for the day. Use any veggies you want, but I like bell peppers, corn, and purple cauliflower florets. This is an awesome dinner if you have veggies and chicken you need to use up fast. If you crave sour cream, opt for coconut cream instead. Add a dollop to the bowl and dive in! Scoop on some salsa and it may remind you of a certain burrito bowl from a certain restaurant, but without all the added sodium.

Serves: 4 to 6

1 tablespoon coconut oil
2 boneless skinless chicken
   breasts, cubed
1 medium red onion, chopped
2 bell peppers, any color or a
   mix, cored and sliced
2 cups fresh corn kernels
1 head purple cauliflower,
   cut into florets
Sea salt
Freshly ground black pepper
Full-fat coconut cream, for
   serving (optional)

1. In a skillet over medium-high heat, heat the coconut oil.

2. Add the chicken to the skillet, followed by the red onion. Reduce the heat to medium and sauté until the chicken begins to brown, about 5 minutes.

3. Add the bell peppers, corn, and purple cauliflower. Sauté for 10 minutes until everything is cooked thoroughly. Season with sea salt and pepper. Serve topped with coconut cream (if using).

> **VARIATION TIP:** Serve this filling stuffed into Cauliflower Tortillas (page 139) for a real fajita experience. Add salsa and guacamole for topping.

Chinese Chicken Salad

Prep time: 15 minutes / Total time: 15 minutes

Chinese chicken salad is one of my favorite dishes, but it tends to have loads of sodium and unnecessary additives. My spin on this popular dish will save you from ordering out, and you can easily make it at home for a Friday movie night in a jiff. This Chinese chicken salad is oh so flavorful and has an interesting twist—fresh ginger—that boosts antioxidants and helps fight inflammation.

Serves: 4 to 6

For the dressing

2 cups freshly squeezed lemon juice
1 cup freshly squeezed lime juice
1 cup coconut aminos

For the Chinese chicken salad

2 cups shredded precooked chicken
4 cups shredded coleslaw mix (red and green cabbage and carrots)
1 cup raw cashews
2 tablespoons grated peeled fresh ginger
½ cup chopped fresh cilantro (optional)

To make the dressing

In a medium bowl, whisk the lemon juice, lime juice, and coconut aminos. Set aside.

To make the Chinese chicken salad

1. Place the chicken in a large bowl.

2. Add the coleslaw mix and cashews.

3. Sprinkle with the ginger and top with the cilantro (if using).

4. Pour the dressing over the salad and toss to combine.

INGREDIENT TIP: Peel fresh ginger with a spoon. The skin peels off easily and you won't waste as much that way.

Chicken Burgers

Prep time: 15 minutes / Cook time: 10 minutes / Total time: 25 minutes

I'm a huge burger fan. Seriously. I ask my hubby to make them multiple times per week in summer. I love burgers because they are easy, can be loaded with veggies, and are filling because of the high protein content. These chicken burgers do not disappoint. We add bacon for an even more powerful protein boost. Make these for the family tonight!

Serves: 4 to 6

1 pound organic free-range
    ground chicken
1 medium red onion, chopped
½ cup chopped fresh tarragon
Sea salt
Freshly ground black pepper
4 to 6 large iceberg lettuce leaves
1 medium tomato, sliced

1. In a bowl, mix the ground chicken, red onion, and tarragon. Season with sea salt and pepper. Mix again to combine. Form the chicken mixture into 4 to 6 patties.

2. Place a cast iron skillet over medium-high heat. When hot, add the chicken patties. Cook for 5 to 10 minutes, turning once, or until they are no longer pink in the middle.

3. Serve the chicken patties wrapped in the lettuce leaves and topped with the tomato.

SERVING TIP: Halve 4 to 6 medium sweet potatoes lengthwise and bake them on a baking sheet that has been sprayed with cooking oil in a preheated 375°F oven for about 30 minutes. Use these as "buns" for the burgers. Top with Simple Ketchup (page 127) and/or Home-made Mayonnaise (page 126).

VARIATION TIP: Turn your chicken burger into a chicken club: Wrap the patties in iceberg lettuce leaves. Add 2 cooked bacon slices, 1 grilled eggplant slice, 1 grilled onion slice, 1 tomato slice, and a drizzle of Paleo Ranch Dressing (page 137) for the ultimate in deliciousness without all the carbs.

Chicken Bruschetta

Prep time: 20 minutes / **Cook time:** 20 minutes / **Total time:** 40 minutes

Missing bruschetta while eating Paleo? It's all good because this is the perfect transition recipe for you. Instead of using bread, I use chicken breast and it works wonderfully! This healthy recipe will cool you down on hot summer nights. The tomatoes and fresh basil are refreshing. Drizzle with extra-virgin olive oil and wash them down with a nice glass of wine and you are set for the weekend.

Serves: 4 to 6

2 cups finely diced tomato
1 medium onion, diced
1 cup chopped fresh basil, plus
　 a few leaves for garnishing
2 tablespoons chopped garlic
6 tablespoons EVOO, divided
¼ cup balsamic vinegar
Sea salt
Freshly ground black pepper
4 to 6 boneless skinless
　 chicken breasts

1. Preheat the oven to 350°F.

2. In a medium bowl, combine the tomato, onion, basil, garlic, 2 tablespoons of EVOO, and the vinegar. Season with sea salt and pepper. Stir to combine and let marinate for 10 to 15 minutes, or longer for a more vibrant flavor.

3. While the bruschetta topping marinates, in a skillet over medium-high heat, heat 2 tablespoons of EVOO. Place the chicken breasts in the skillet. Sear each side for 4 minutes. Cook for about 5 minutes more, turning the chicken occasionally, until nicely browned on the outside and just cooked through. If this chicken starts to get too brown, lower the heat. Remove the chicken from the skillet and set aside to cool.

4. Place the cooled chicken in a baking dish and layer the tomato mixture on top.

5. Bake for 10 minutes. Serve warm, drizzled with the remaining 2 tablespoons of EVOO and garnished with basil leaves.

> VARIATION TIP: If you're tired of chicken, substitute thick-cut boneless pork chops.

Coconut-Chicken Nuggets

Prep time: 10 minutes / Cook time: 50 minutes / Total time: 1 hour

Chicken nuggets are an easy weeknight meal, but not always the healthiest option. Make this updated Paleo version instead. These nuggets are made with coconut oil and coated with crispy shredded coconut. They are easy to make and taste so amazing you won't miss traditional chicken nuggets ever again. I promise!

Serves: 4 to 6

2 cups unsweetened
    shredded coconut
2 tablespoons garlic powder
Sea salt
Freshly ground black pepper
1 cup coconut oil
4 to 6 boneless skinless
    chicken breasts, cubed

1. Preheat the oven to 350°F. Line a baking sheet with parchment paper and set aside.

2. In a medium bowl, stir together the shredded coconut and garlic powder. Season with sea salt and pepper. Mix again to combine.

3. Place the coconut oil in a shallow bowl. Add the chicken and turn to coat. Dip the oiled chicken in the coconut mixture, coating both sides evenly. Place the chicken nuggets on the prepared baking sheet.

4. Bake for 40 to 50 minutes until golden and crispy.

VARIATION TIP: For added flavor, stir chopped fresh herbs (thyme, oregano, or cilantro) into the coconut mixture before coating the chicken chunks.

Chicken & Veggie Grill Packs

Prep time: 10 minutes / Cook time: 40 minutes / Total time: 50 minutes

Heat up your grill, grab some aluminum foil, and let's make chicken and veggie grill packs! These are great on warm nights when you don't want to turn on the oven, and you can fill the packs with any spices you like. Feel free to add more than what's listed here because the more flavor in these chicken and veggie grill packs, the better!

Serves: 4 to 6

½ pound boneless skinless
   chicken breast, cubed
2 zucchini, sliced
1 medium red onion, sliced
1 pound asparagus, woody ends
   removed and discarded
4 bell peppers, a mix of colors,
   cored and sliced
2 garlic cloves, chopped
2 tablespoons EVOO
2 tablespoons balsamic vinegar
Sea salt (optional)
Freshly ground black pepper (optional)

1. Preheat the grill to medium-high heat.

2. Tear off 4 to 6 large pieces of aluminum foil. Evenly divide the chicken, zucchini, red onion, asparagus, bell peppers, and garlic among the foil pieces. Drizzle with EVOO and vinegar. Season with sea salt and pepper, if desired. Wrap the chicken and veggies in the foil and fold it over to seal, forming grill packs (see tip).

3. Place the packs on the grill. Close the lid and grill for 30 to 40 minutes, or until the chicken is cooked through.

PRO TIP: When wrapping up your foil packets, be sure to leave a bit of space inside so there is room for steam to circulate around the food and cook it evenly.

Chicken Pineapple Skewers

Prep time: 10 minutes / **Cook time:** 30 minutes / **Total time:** 40 minutes

Chicken and pineapple is one of the best combos ever. These chicken skewers grill up fast and freeze well. If you want to freeze these as a make-ahead meal, do not cook anything. Simply skewer all the ingredients, wrap them in aluminum foil, and freeze. When you are ready to cook, remove the skewers from the freezer to thaw; once thawed, just grill.

Serves: 4 to 6

1½ pounds boneless skinless chicken breast, cubed (see tip)

4 bell peppers, any color or a mix, cut into squares

1 medium red onion, cut into squares

1 head garlic, cloves separated and peeled

1 pineapple, cored and sliced

1. Preheat a grill to medium-high heat.

2. Using 8 to 10 skewers, place one piece of chicken on each skewer, followed by a piece of bell pepper, a square of red onion, a garlic clove, and a pineapple slice. Repeat until the skewers are full.

3. Wrap the skewers in aluminum foil. Place the wrapped skewers on the grill. Cook for 20 to 30 minutes until the chicken is thoroughly cooked through and the pineapple is caramelized.

> **PRO TIP:** Cut the chicken into regularly sized cubes so they cook evenly, and make the cubes as large as possible to prevent them from overcooking and drying out.

Turkey-Stuffed Bell Peppers

Prep time: 10 minutes / Cook time: 35 minutes / Total time: 45 minutes

Ground turkey is fantastic because it's lean and very flavorful if you spice it correctly. This recipe is awesome if you have bell peppers starting to wrinkle in the fridge. Use coconut cream as a topping instead of sour cream and get ready to enjoy perfect Paleo stuffed bell peppers.

Serves: 4 to 6

1 pound ground turkey
1 medium red onion, diced
1 tablespoon chopped garlic
¼ cup chopped fresh oregano leaves
Sea salt
Freshly ground black pepper
6 bell peppers, any color or a
    mix, stemmed and seeded
½ cup finely chopped fresh
    cilantro (optional)
Full-fat coconut cream, for
    serving (optional)

1. Preheat the oven to 425°F. Line a large baking dish with parchment paper and set aside.

2. In a skillet over medium heat, combine the turkey, red onion, garlic, and oregano. Season with sea salt and pepper. Cook for about 5 minutes, stirring to break up the meat, until the turkey is browned.

3. Stand the bell peppers in the prepared baking dish.

4. Carefully spoon the ground turkey mixture into each bell pepper.

5. Bake for 30 minutes, or until each bell pepper is nice and crispy.

6. Serve topped with fresh cilantro and coconut cream (if using).

VARIATION TIP: Use any type of meat you like here, including ground beef, bacon, or sausage.

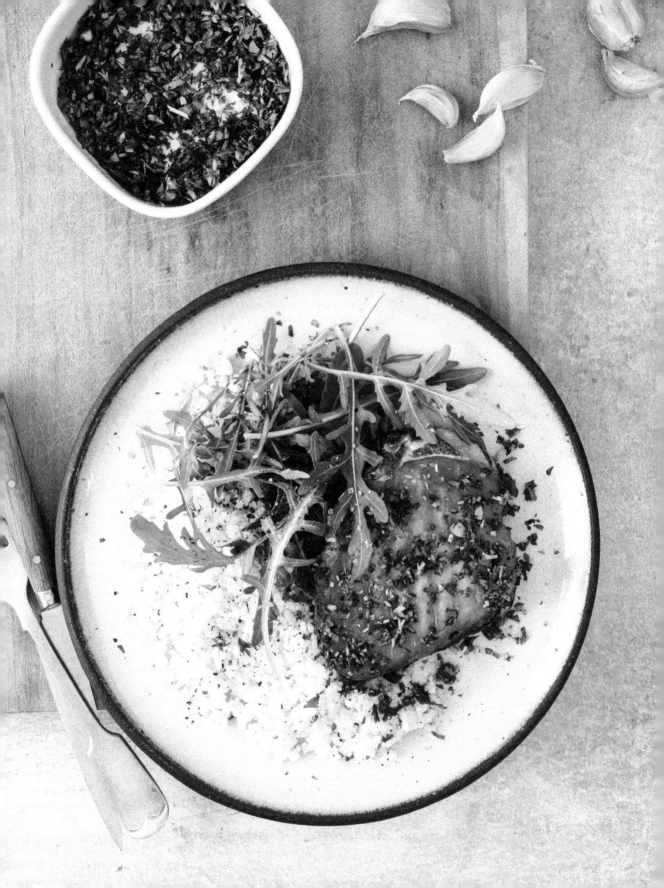

Beef & Pork Mains

Opposite: Garlic & Herb Pork Chops, page 103

Taco-Stuffed Sweet Potatoes

Prep time: 5 minutes / **Cook time:** 45 minutes / **Total time:** 50 minutes

Taco-stuffed sweet potatoes are a staple meal in any Paleo diet. They are fairly easy to make and satisfy that taco craving. Once ready, slice open your sweet potatoes halfway so you can fill them with all that taco goodness.

Serves: 4 to 6

4 to 6 sweet potatoes
1½ pounds organic ground beef
1 medium red onion, diced, plus more for serving
¼ cup taco seasoning
1 cup salsa, for serving

1. Preheat the oven to 375°F.

2. Wrap each sweet potato in aluminum foil. Poke holes in the foil so the sweet potatoes cook properly. Bake for about 40 to 45 minutes until soft.

3. In a skillet over medium heat, cook the ground beef for 5 to 7 minutes, stirring to break up the meat, until mostly browned.

4. Add the red onion and taco seasoning. Stir to combine and continue cooking until the beef is done, about 5 minutes more.

5. Slice open the sweet potatoes about halfway. Fill each sweet potato with the ground beef mixture.

6. Top with salsa and dig in.

> **VARIATION TIP:** Add butter lettuce, coconut cream, guacamole, and chopped fresh cilantro as taco toppings for extra flavor and texture.

Beef & Broccoli

Prep time: 10 minutes / Cook time: 15 minutes / Total time: 25 minutes

Beef and broccoli is delicious, but can be made with tons of sodium. Using coconut aminos instead of the traditional salty soy sauce lightens the sodium amount and gives this dish a less salty taste. Flank steak is a leaner meat, but still packs the protein.

Serves: 4 to 6

1½ pounds flank steak, thinly sliced
¼ cup coconut aminos
3 garlic cloves, minced
2 tablespoons minced
   peeled fresh ginger
4 cups broccoli florets
Sea salt
Freshly ground black pepper

1. In a skillet over medium heat, sauté the flank steak for 3 to 5 minutes.

2. Add the coconut aminos and garlic. Sauté everything for 2 to 3 minutes until the beef is slightly browned.

3. Add the ginger and broccoli. Sauté for 4 to 5 minutes more until cooked through. Season with sea salt and pepper.

VARIATION TIP: Serve this over a bed of cauliflower rice, garnished with sliced scallions. It'll quash any cravings you've been having for your favorite Chinese takeout.

Pork & Veggie Shish Kabobs

Prep time: 10 minutes / **Cook time:** 30 minutes / **Total time:** 40 minutes

These kabobs can be prepped ahead and stashed in the freezer until you are ready to bake them. Chop your veggies into chunky pieces so they cook well.

Serves: 4 to 6

1½ pounds pork tenderloin, cubed

3 bell peppers, any color or a
    mix, chopped into chunks

1 medium red onion,
    chopped into chunks

1 pineapple, cored and
    chopped into chunks

1 head garlic, cloves
    separated and peeled

1. Preheat the oven to 350°F.

2. Take 10 to 12 skewers and thread each with a piece of pork, a piece of bell pepper, a piece of red onion, a pineapple chunk, and a garlic clove. Repeat with the remaining ingredients to fill the skewers. Wrap the skewers in aluminum foil and place on a baking sheet.

3. Bake for 25 to 30 minutes until browned and crispy.

VARIATION TIP: Add other veggies—mushrooms, cherry tomatoes, or thickly sliced zucchini rounds—to the skewers for more color and flavor.

Steak & Pepper Fajitas

Prep time: 10 minutes / Cook time: 20 minutes / Total time: 30 minutes

I know when I think of fajitas I think of a delicious steak and pepper combo. The best steak to use is flank steak because it's low in fat and slices very thinly.

Serves: 4 to 6

1 pound flank steak, thinly sliced
2 cups sliced bell pepper,
    any color or a mix
1 cup diced red onion
2 tablespoons chopped garlic
Sea salt
Freshly ground black pepper
1 avocado, halved, pitted, and diced
1 cup chopped fresh cilantro
1 lime, cut into wedges

1. In a skillet over medium-high heat, sauté the flank steak for 3 to 6 minutes.

2. Add the bell pepper, red onion, and garlic. Sauté for 5 to 10 minutes until everything is cooked through. Season with sea salt and pepper.

3. Serve topped with avocado, cilantro, and lime wedges.

> VARIATION TIP: For a truer fajita experience, serve as a filling for Cauliflower Tortillas [page 139]. Add coconut cream, salsa, and guacamole for topping.

Beef Chili

Prep time: 10 minutes / Cook time: 6 hours 10 minutes / Total time: 6 hours 20 minutes

People think when they go Paleo, they can't have chili; just swap the beans for sweet potatoes.

Serves: 4 to 6

1½ pounds organic ground beef
1 (28-ounce) can organic diced
  tomatoes, with their juice
6 garlic cloves, minced
1 medium red onion, chopped
3 cups chopped sweet potatoes
2 tablespoons chili powder
Sea salt
Freshly ground black pepper

1. In a skillet over medium heat, cook the ground beef for 5 to 10 minutes, stirring occasionally to break up the meat, until browned. Transfer the beef to a slow cooker.

2. Add the tomatoes along with their juice, the garlic, red onion, sweet potatoes, and chili powder. Season with sea salt and pepper.

3. Cover the cooker and set to high heat. Cook for at least 6 hours. The longer you cook the chili, the better it tastes.

VARIATION TIP: Make a big pot of this chili to serve a crowd. You can extend it by adding additional veggies—such as corn, bell peppers, more tomatoes, or mushrooms—without emptying your wallet. Just be sure to boost the garlic, onion, and chili powder, too, so it still has plenty of flavor.

Garlic & Herb Pork Chops

Prep time: 5 minutes / Cook time: 25 minutes / Total time: 30 minutes

Pork is a delicious light meat, and a wonder for Paleo diets because it's a light protein option that cooks quickly. It also freezes well. Prep the pork chops by rubbing them with ghee, minced garlic, and onion, and stash them in the freezer until you are ready to use them.

Serves: 4 to 6

4 to 6 bone-in pork chops
2 tablespoons ghee
4 garlic cloves, minced
2 tablespoons minced fresh
  oregano leaves
½ cup chopped fresh cilantro, minced
½ cup chopped fresh parsley, minced

1. Preheat the oven to 375°F.

2. Place the pork chops on a baking sheet and rub ghee all over each chop. Top each chop with garlic and oregano.

3. Bake for 20 to 25 minutes until browned and cooked through.

4. Serve topped with cilantro and parsley.

VARIATION TIP: Make this with lamb chops instead of pork. Substitute fresh mint for the oregano as lamb and mint are such a great match.

Grilled Pineapple Pork Chops

Prep time: 10 minutes / **Cook time:** 10 minutes / **Total time:** 20 minutes

There is a reason pork and pineapple go so well together. The two flavors combined bring out the best in each other. The nice thing about adding pineapple to pork is that the pineapple adds a level of sweetness without being overbearing. For this recipe you'll need one whole pineapple, peeled, cored, and sliced. You'll also need a grill.

Serves: 4 to 6

1 cup honey
4 cups Barbecue Sauce (page 132), with a little bit reserved for serving
4 to 6 bone-in pork chops
2 tablespoons minced peeled fresh ginger
2 garlic cloves, minced
1 whole pineapple, peeled, cored, and sliced

1. Preheat the grill to high heat.

2. In a small bowl, stir together the honey and barbecue sauce. Brush the pork chops with the sauce. Rub the ginger and garlic onto the chops, pressing it to adhere to the sauce. Place the chops on the grill.

3. Top the pork chops with the fresh pineapple slices, or place them directly on the grill. Grill for 4 to 5 minutes per side until browned. If the pineapple starts to burn, move it to a cooler portion of the grill.

4. Once the pork chops are done, drizzle with more barbecue sauce.

> INGREDIENT TIP: When buying pork chops for grilling, try to get center-cut rib chops. This cut is slightly more fatty than other cuts, making it an ideal choice for juicy, delicious grilled chops.

Pork & Sautéed Apples

Prep time: 5 minutes / **Cook time:** 15 minutes / **Total time:** 20 minutes

Pork and apples go together like Pooh Bear and honey. There is a comfort that goes along with having pork and apples for dinner. The apples complement the pork and everything hits your taste buds in this fantastic, harmonious flavor. Leave the skins on the apples and don't worry about overcooking them. You want them to be nice and soft and cooked well with the cinnamon. The pork chops will brown pretty fast, so be careful not to overcook them.

Serves: 4 to 6

2 tablespoons ghee
1 cup diced red onion
4 to 6 bone-in pork chops
4 cups diced unpeeled
   Granny Smith apples
1 tablespoon ground cinnamon
Sea salt
Freshly ground black pepper

1. In a skillet over medium-high heat, heat the ghee. Add the red onion. Cook for 3 to 4 minutes until it begins to soften.

2. Place the pork chops in the skillet. Cook for 2 to 3 minutes per side.

3. Add the apples and sprinkle with the cinnamon. Season with sea salt and pepper. Cook for 5 minutes more until everything is thoroughly cooked. If the pan gets too dry, add a splash of water.

VARIATION TIP: To make this a one-pot meal, remove the pork chops from the skillets once they are well seared on each side, and set aside. Add a small head of green cabbage, thinly sliced, to the skillet along with the apples. Cook, stirring occasionally, until the cabbage is tender. Return the pork chops to the skillet and cook for 1 to 2 minutes more until the pork is heated and cooked through.

Bacon-Wrapped Asparagus

Prep time: 10 minutes / Cook time: 25 minutes / Total time: 35 minutes

Bacon-wrapped asparagus is one of those recipes that can be used as an appetizer or as a meal. Asparagus is so good for you! Some people don't like it because of the way it makes them "smell" but, truth be told, it is loaded with folate, fiber, vitamins A, C, E, and K, as well as chromium. Think of asparagus as the super veggie, because that's what it is!

Serves: 4 to 6

1 pound fresh asparagus, woody
   ends removed and discarded
2 tablespoons EVOO
1 pound nitrate-free bacon
5 garlic cloves, minced
2 tablespoons fresh oregano leaves
1 cup chopped fresh cilantro

1. Preheat the oven to 350°F.

2. Lay the asparagus on a baking sheet and brush it with EVOO.

3. Wrap a slice of uncooked bacon around each asparagus spear.

4. Sprinkle the garlic and oregano over the wrapped asparagus.

5. Bake for 20 to 25 minutes until the bacon is nice and crispy.

6. Garnish with fresh cilantro and enjoy!

> VARIATION TIP: Try making this with long-stemmed broccoli florets or large, halved Brussels sprouts (you might want to halve the bacon strips, depending on how large the sprouts are).

Apple & Sausage–Stuffed Squash

Prep time: 5 minutes / **Cook time:** 1 hour 5 minutes / **Total time:** 1 hour 10 minutes

Squash is such an amazing veggie and, sadly, most people only use it during fall. And, while this recipe will bring you straight into autumn, you can make it any time of year.

Serves: 4 to 6

Coconut oil spray, for preparing
   the baking sheet
2 to 3 acorn squashes, halved
1½ pounds nitrate-free ground sausage
2 cups diced apple
1 cup diced red onion
Sea salt
Freshly ground black pepper

1. Preheat the oven to 400°F. Coat a rimmed baking sheet with coconut oil spray.

2. Place the halved acorn squashes, cut-side up, on the prepared sheet. Bake for 1 hour, or until the squash is nice and crispy. Set aside.

3. In a skillet over medium heat, cook the sausage and red onion for 3 to 5 minutes, until browned. Using a slotted spoon, transfer the sausage and red onion to a medium bowl.

4. Add the apple to the sausage and red onion mixture. Stir to combine. Spoon the sausage mixture into the acorn squash halves, filling them, and place them back on the baking sheet.

5. Bake for an additional 5 minutes until everything is nice and crispy.

6. Season with sea salt and pepper.

> INGREDIENT TIP: Acorn squash are large enough that one, filled with the sausage and apple mixture, can easily feed two people. To make smaller one-serving squash boats, use 4 to 6 delicata squash. The great thing about delicata is you can eat the skin, too.

Sweet Potato Bacon Avocado Salsa Bites

Prep time: 10 minutes / Cook time: 30 minutes / Total time: 40 minutes

Sweet potatoes and avocados for dinner? Yes, please! The two make a great combo, especially paired with fresh cilantro and salsa. Add crumbled bacon bits and you've got yourself a winning meal! This recipe can be prepped ahead, if desired. Just add freshly squeezed lemon juice to the avocados so they stay nice and green. Prep the sweet potatoes the night before by cleaning them and slicing.

Serves: 4 to 6

1 pound nitrate-free bacon
2 cups diced avocado
2 cups fresh salsa
1 cup minced fresh cilantro,
    2 tablespoons reserved
    for garnishing
6 sweet potatoes, unpeeled
    and thinly sliced
2 tablespoons EVOO
Sea salt
Freshly ground black pepper
2 tablespoons freshly
    squeezed lime juice

1. Preheat the oven to 450°F.

2. In a skillet over medium heat, cook the bacon for about 5 minutes until crispy. Transfer to paper towels to drain. Chop the bacon into small bits.

3. In a medium bowl, mash together the avocado, salsa, and cilantro until smooth. Stash the avo-salsa in the fridge until ready to use.

4. Place the sliced sweet potatoes on a baking sheet. Drizzle with EVOO and sprinkle with sea salt and pepper.

5. Bake for 20 to 25 minutes until crispy.

6. Top the cooked sweet potato slices with the avo-salsa, sprinkle with lime juice, and scatter bacon bits and fresh cilantro over the top.

VARIATION TIP: Turn these into full-fledged Paleo nachos by adding pickled jalapeño rings and sliced olives on top.

Bacon Pork Tenderloin

Prep time: 10 minutes / Cook time: 30 minutes / Total time: 40 minutes

This bacon and pork tenderloin will be a weeknight repeat in your house. It's easy to prepare, kiddos love it, and it's wrapped in bacon. What more could you possibly want from a pork recipe? We make our own rub here, but use a good store-bought one, if you prefer. Serve with a heaping side of veggies.

Serves: 4 to 6

2 teaspoons paprika
1 teaspoon chili powder
1 teaspoon ground cinnamon
Sea salt
Freshly ground black pepper
1 pork tenderloin (about 1 pound)
1 cup EVOO
1 pound nitrate-free bacon

1. Preheat the oven to 350°F.

2. In a small bowl, stir together the paprika, chili powder, and cinnamon. Season with sea salt and pepper. Stir again to combine.

3. Rub the pork tenderloin all over with the EVOO. Sprinkle on the spice mixture and rub it into the pork (see tip).

4. Wrap the pork tenderloin with the bacon strips and place the tenderloin on a baking sheet.

5. Bake for 25 to 30 minutes until the tenderloin is cooked through (145°F on an instant-read thermometer). Remove from the oven and tent with aluminum foil. Let rest for 10 minutes before slicing and serving.

PREPARATION TIP: To make the pork especially tender and flavorful, refrigerate for up to 24 hours after applying the spice mixture.

Bacon-Wrapped Meatballs

Prep time: 15 minutes / **Cook time:** 35 minutes / **Total time:** 50 minutes

Bacon-wrapped anything is delicious, but wrap meatballs in bacon and zucchini and you've got yourself one amazing meal. Use a spiralizer to slice the zucchini and be prepared for a recipe that you'll come back to often. Bonus: This recipe also makes a great appetizer for last-minute parties.

Serves: 4 to 6

1 pound organic ground beef
1 medium red onion, diced
2 garlic cloves, minced
¼ cup coconut aminos
2 cups spiralized zucchini zoodles
1 (12-ounce) package
   nitrate-free bacon

1. Preheat the oven to 350°F.

2. In a medium bowl, combine the ground beef, red onion, garlic, and coconut aminos. Mix everything until combined. Roll the meat mixture into 1- to 2-inch meatballs.

3. Carefully wrap a zucchini zoodle around each meatball. Wrap a bacon slice around the zucchini-wrapped meatballs and secure with a toothpick. Put the prepared meatballs on a baking sheet.

4. Bake for 30 to 35 minutes until cooked through.

> **INGREDIENT TIP:** Use ground turkey or ground lamb, if you prefer, instead of the beef.

Paleo Beef Bowls

Prep time: 5 minutes / Cook time: 10 minutes / Total time: 15 minutes

This is probably the easiest recipe in this entire book. It's wonderful for nights when you don't feel like cooking and can literally be made with whatever you have in your fridge. It's great, too, for using those veggies about to go bad, and it can be whipped up at the last minute. You will be the hero of your household because you will have dinner on the table and ready to go in under 20 minutes. It's okay; you can thank me later.

Serves: 4 to 6

1½ pounds organic ground beef
2 cups chopped red onion
1 cup sliced cherry tomatoes
2 cups broccoli florets
2 cups sliced bell peppers,
    any color or a mix
Sea salt
Freshly ground black pepper

1. In a skillet over medium heat, combine the ground beef and red onion. Sauté for about 5 minutes, stirring to break up the meat, until it begins to brown.

2. Add the cherry tomatoes, broccoli, and bell peppers. Sauté for 5 minutes more. You want the veggies to be slightly crisp, so don't overcook them. Transfer to serving bowls. Season with sea salt and pepper.

VARIATION TIP: Serve topped with Homemade Mayonnaise [page 126], guacamole, or salsa.

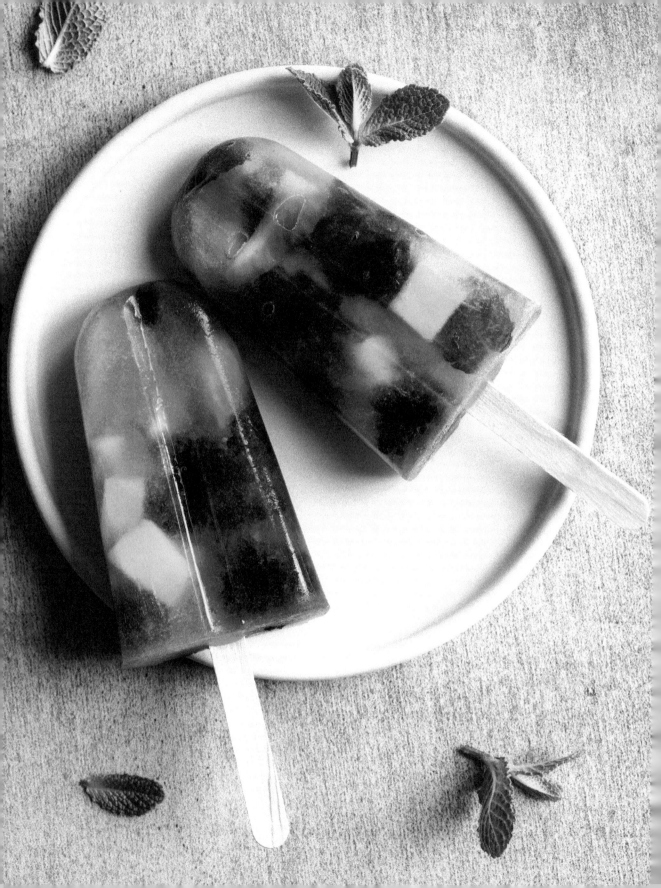

8

Desserts

Opposite: Fruity Ice Pops, page 118

Banana-Coconut Ice Cream

Prep time: 15 minutes, plus overnight freezing of the bananas / **Freezing time:** 2 hours

Total time: 2 hours 15 minutes, plus overnight freezing

Yes, ice cream and Paleo can go together. Not only is this ice cream healthy, but it's also one of the creamiest ice creams you'll ever have. And it's made with just two main ingredients: bananas and coconut milk. You don't even have to use the coconut milk if you don't want to, but I find it lends even more creaminess to the texture. Top with cacao nibs for a banana-chocolate treat. You will need to freeze your bananas overnight before completing this recipe.

Serves: 4 to 6

3 ripe bananas, peeled, thinly
   sliced, and frozen overnight
   in a glass container

2 cups almond-coconut milk

1 cup unsweetened shredded coconut

1 cup fresh strawberries,
   sliced (optional)

1 cup cacao nibs

1. In a high-powered blender, combine the frozen bananas and almond-coconut milk. Blend on medium speed. At first the bananas will look like they aren't turning into ice cream, but have patience and keep blending; they'll turn into ice cream after about 3 minutes.

2. Transfer the ice cream into a glass container with a lid. Cover and freeze for at least 2 hours.

3. Once frozen, serve in sundae glasses topped with shredded coconut, strawberry slices (if using), and cacao nibs.

> **VARIATION TIP:** For a chocolatey version, add ¼ teaspoon of vanilla extract and 3 tablespoons of unsweetened cocoa powder along with the bananas and almond-coconut milk.

Apple Pie Baked Apples

Prep time: 15 minutes / Cook time: 30 minutes / Total time: 45 minutes

Crave apple pie? Me, too—and not just on Thanksgiving. This is a tasty way to use up leftover apples lying around. Keep the tops of the apples after you remove them. You'll use them to top the baked apples.

Serves: 4 to 6

6 large apples (any variety;
   I suggest using different varieties,
   especially for kiddos!)
1 cup pecans, chopped
⅓ cup honey
1 tablespoon ground cinnamon
1 tablespoon vanilla extract

1. Preheat the oven to 375°F. Line a baking sheet with parchment paper and set aside.

2. Cut off the tops of each apple, reserving them, and spoon out the core.

3. Carefully remove the remaining apple insides, being careful not to break the apple skin, and finely dice.

4. In a medium bowl, combine the diced apple, pecans, honey, cinnamon, and vanilla. Fill each hollowed-out apple skin with the apple mixture. Cover each apple with its reserved top. Place the filled apples on the prepared baking sheet.

5. Bake for 20 to 30 minutes, or until the apples are nice and crispy.

> VARIATION TIP: Serve these topped with whipped coconut cream for an especially festive dessert.

Paleo Peanut Butter Cups

Prep time: 15 minutes / **Freezing time:** 2 hours / **Total time:** 2 hours 15 minutes

For this recipe, you'll need peanut butter cup molds or mini muffin tins. These treats are great with a cup of black coffee. Your chocolate cravings will also thank you as these little bites of heaven work well for a quick pick-me-up and as a yummy dessert!

Serves: 4 to 6

2 cups unsweetened cacao powder
1 cup almond butter
1 cup coconut oil, melted
2 teaspoons vanilla extract
1 cup peanut butter
Chunky sea salt

1. In a blender, combine the cacao powder, almond butter, melted coconut oil, and vanilla. Blend until smooth. Slowly fill each peanut butter cup mold about halfway with the mixture.

2. Place a scoop of peanut butter into the middle of each mold.

3. Cover the peanut butter with more of the chocolate-almond butter mixture to fill the molds.

4. Sprinkle each cup with chunky sea salt. Place the molds into the freezer and let set for at least 2 hours, and preferably overnight.

> VARIATION TIP: Add texture and flavor by sprinkling unsweetened shredded coconut on top of the second layer of chocolate-almond butter before chilling.

Fruit Shish Kabobs

Prep time: 20 minutes / Total time: 20 minutes

I love fruit and I tend to buy it in bulk, but my husband doesn't really eat it much, so I'm left with tons I can't finish on my own. This is why I love fruit shish kabobs. If you really want to amp up this recipe, grill the kabobs for an even more satisfying treat. So go on, take this book into your kitchen and let's use up that leftover fruit!

Makes: 4 to 6 skewers

1 pound organic strawberries,
 tops removed
1 whole pineapple, cored and sliced
6 peaches, sliced
6 apples, sliced
1 pound coconut chunks

1. Take a strawberry and place it at the bottom of a skewer. Add a pineapple slice, a peach slice, an apple slice, and lastly a coconut chunk. Repeat until all the ingredients are skewered.

2. Keep refrigerated in an airtight container for up to 5 days.

VARIATION TIP: If you want to take these skewers to the next level, preheat a grill to medium-low heat. Place the kebobs on the grill and grill for 5 to 10 minutes, turning, until warmed and slightly charred, or to your liking.

Fruity Ice Pops

Prep time: 10 minutes / **Freezing time:** 4 hours / **Total time:** 4 hours 10 minutes

It's a scorcher outside. Need a way to cool off? Make these delicious fruity ice pops and stash the extras in the freezer. All you need are coconut water, ice pop molds, and fresh fruit. No need to waste money at the store buying ice pops full of sugar, food dyes, and who knows how many additives. Make these tonight with any leftover fruit you have in your house and enjoy them tomorrow!

Serves: 4 to 6; makes about 12 ice pops

2 cups coconut water
2 cups sliced fresh
   strawberries, divided
1 cup fresh blueberries
1 mango, diced
½ cup fresh mint leaves

1. In a blender, combine the coconut water and 1½ cups of strawberries. Blend until smooth.

2. Fill each ice pop mold about halfway, dividing the remaining ½ cup of sliced strawberries, the blueberries, and the mango among them.

3. Carefully place the fresh mint leaves into the molds around the fruit.

4. Fill each mold with the strawberry-coconut water mixture.

5. Insert the handles and freeze the molds for at least 4 hours, or until frozen.

> **VARIATION TIP:** For a creamy version, use half coconut water and half coconut milk.

Easy Coconut Fat Balls

Prep time: 20 minutes / **Freezing time:** 2 hours / **Total time:** 2 hours 20 minutes

Have a sweet craving? These coconut fat balls will beckon you to the fridge without the guilt. These little protein powerhouses pack a whopping 25 grams of protein per three balls. They make a fantastic snack before that weightlifting workout or right after that long trail run when you need something quick and easy. They are also great just before you head into the grocery store so you don't shop hungry, because we all know how awful that is—I just end up buying a bunch of food I don't actually need. This way, I'm full and buy only what's on my list.

Makes: Approximately 48 balls

1 cup unsweetened shredded coconut
1 cup walnuts
¼ cup almond butter
2 teaspoons ground cinnamon
1 cup coconut oil

1. Line a rimmed baking sheet with parchment paper and set aside.

2. In a food processor, combine the shredded coconut, walnuts, almond butter, and cinnamon. Pulse until finely ground.

3. Add the coconut oil. Pulse until a dough forms. Remove the dough from the processor. Roll the dough into 1-inch balls and place on the prepared baking sheet. Freeze for at least 2 hours.

4. Keep frozen in a sealed glass container for up to 2 weeks.

> PRO TIP: Use a small cookie scoop to form the balls. It will save time and make uniformly sized balls.

Apple Almond Butter Bites

Prep time: 20 minutes / **Total time:** 20 minutes

There is something about sliced apples with peanut butter that brings up a lot of fond child-hood memories. My mom used to make these for me so I would have a healthy snack at school. It's something I've carried into my adult years and a snack I continue to make for my children. This delicious recipe gives your body the energy boost it needs. You get a ton of protein from the nuts and a creamy rich taste from the nut butter. To top it off, there's the hint of sweetness from the apples. This works as the perfect, healthy snack, but also serves as a wonderful late-night treat!

Serves: 4 to 6

6 apples, cored and thinly sliced
1 (12-ounce) jar almond butter
    or peanut butter
2 cups unsalted nuts and seeds (any
    combination of sliced almonds,
    chopped pecans, chopped
    walnuts, pumpkin seeds, etc.)
1 cup unsweetened shredded coconut

1. Spread each apple slice with a thin layer of nut butter.

2. Top each slice with some nuts and seeds.

3. Sprinkle the shredded coconut over the apple slices and enjoy. These apple slices will keep, refrigerated in an airtight glass container, for up to 3 days.

> **PRO TIP:** Before spreading the nut butter on the apple slices, squeeze some fresh lemon juice over them to keep them from browning.

Banana Coconut Split

Prep time: 10 minutes / **Total time:** 10 minutes

If you like banana splits, then you are going to love this healthy amped-up version. And don't worry about post-sugar hangover or dessert food guilt—there is nothing to feel guilty about here. These power banana splits have healthy fats and protein, and provide an antioxidant boost. You could even eat this gem for breakfast, and it makes a wonderful after-school snack for hungry kiddos. Bananas are loaded with potassium, which our bodies need. In fact, most people are lacking in their daily recommended amount of potassium, so eat those bananas—especially on hot days! Potassium helps keep your hydration levels in check and helps your muscles recover faster from workouts.

Serves: 4 to 6

4 to 6 bananas, peeled and
  sliced lengthwise
3 cups fresh berries (sliced
  strawberries, raspberries,
  blueberries, blackberries,
  or a mix)
1 cup full-fat coconut cream
2 cups sliced almonds
½ cup honey

1. Arrange the banana slices in a sundae dish or on a plate, 2 banana slices per sundae.

2. Top with the berries.

3. Drizzle coconut cream on top of the banana splits.

4. Sprinkle with the almonds.

5. Drizzle everything with honey and serve.

VARIATION TIP: In place of the honey, top this beauty off with a fresh strawberry sauce. In a saucepan over medium-high heat, stir together ¼ cup of honey and ¼ cup of water. Add 1 cup of sliced fresh strawberries and bring to a boil. Reduce the heat to a simmer and cook for about 5 minutes until the sauce is syrupy. Transfer to a blender and purée until smooth.

Fried Bananas

Prep time: 5 minutes / **Cook time:** 10 minutes / **Total time:** 15 minutes

Have you ever ordered fried bananas for dessert at a restaurant? Heaven, right? They are ooey and gooey and oh so rich tasting. Here, though, instead of whipped cream, I use dairy-free coconut cream, and it's just as delicious as the original. The coconut oil makes these fried bananas even richer—they will literally melt in your mouth. The best part is, you can use bananas that are on their last legs, in fact those will be even tastier fried!

Serves: 4 to 6

1 tablespoon ground cinnamon
½ teaspoon ground nutmeg
⅓ cup coconut oil
¼ cup honey
1 bunch bananas, peeled and quartered
Full-fat coconut cream, for serving (optional)

1. In a small bowl, stir together the cinnamon and nutmeg and set aside.

2. In a skillet over medium-high heat, heat the coconut oil.

3. Pour in the honey and sprinkle the cinnamon-nutmeg mixture into the skillet. Heat until the oil liquefies, 1 to 2 minutes.

4. Carefully place each banana slice into the skillet. Fry for 2 minutes per side until nice and browned. You want the banana slices to be crispy.

5. Drizzle the honey mixture over the top and serve warm with a dollop of coconut cream (if using).

> **VARIATION TIP:** For a different flavor, leave out the cinnamon and nutmeg and add ½ teaspoon of vanilla extract to the honey. Fry the bananas in ghee instead of coconut oil.

Easy Chocolate Pudding

Prep time: 5 minutes / Total time: 15 minutes

Making Paleo-friendly pudding is easier than you think, as long as you have beef gelatin. My favorite brand is Vital Proteins. Invest in beef gelatin; it's worth every single penny. Okay, let's talk about this easy chocolate pudding. Made with avocados and unsweetened cacao powder, you will never go back to store-bought pudding again. Bonus: Your kiddos will love this, too!

Serves: 4 to 6

2 scoops beef gelatin
½ cup melted coconut butter
1 cup unsweetened cacao powder
4 to 6 avocados, pitted and peeled
1 cup honey

1. In a medium bowl, combine the beef gelatin and 1 tablespoon of water. Set aside to let the gelatin bloom. You will know it's blooming when it starts to expand.

2. Add the melted coconut butter and lightly mix everything together. Do not overmix at this stage.

3. Add the cacao powder, avocados, and honey. Stir until it has a pudding-like consistency. Alternatively, use a blender and blend everything together on medium speed until it becomes a pudding. Transfer the pudding to a glass container with a lid and refrigerate for a few hours to firm up. Or, if you can't wait, eat it right after mixing!

> VARIATION TIP: Round out the chocolatey flavor of this pudding by adding 1 teaspoon of vanilla extract along with the honey.

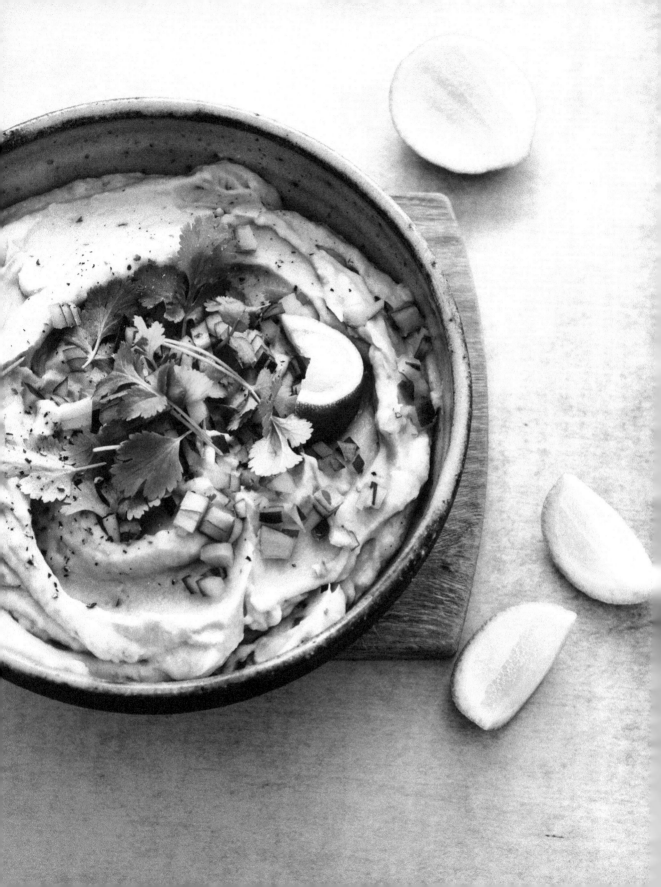

9

Sauces, Dressings & Staples

Opposite: Easy Guacamole, page 138

Homemade Mayonnaise

Prep time: 5 minutes / **Total time:** 10 minutes

Store-bought mayo can be full of sugar, chemicals, and other fillers. This easy homemade mayonnaise can be made faster than going to the store and buying it—and you'll have fresh mayo all week long for all your recipes!

Makes: about 1½ cups;
6 (¼-cup) servings

1 cup avocado oil
2 large eggs
2 teaspoons freshly squeezed lemon
   juice, plus more as needed
½ teaspoon sea salt, plus
   more as needed
1 tablespoon Dijon mustard

1. In a tall jar, combine the avocado oil, eggs, lemon juice, sea salt, and mustard. Using an immersion blender, pulse everything together on medium speed for 1 minute, making sure the blade is placed at the bottom of the jar.

2. Slowly lift the immersion blender to make fluffs in the mayo. Continue this for 2 minutes.

3. Taste and add more lemon juice and sea salt as needed. Transfer to a glass jar with a lid, tightly seal, and refrigerate for up to 4 weeks.

VARIATION TIP: Blend in 1 teaspoon of curry powder for variety.

Simple Ketchup

Prep time: 5 minutes / Total time: 10 minutes

Ketchup is an American diet staple. As good as ketchup is, the problem is, it's full of sugar. It's also typically made with corn syrup. Corn syrup is not good for our bodies as we have a really hard time processing it. It's also been linked to certain cancers. The best way to make home-made ketchup is with minimal, healthy ingredients, such as honey and vinegar. It's also really easy—mix and stir.

Makes: about 1½ cups;
6 (¼-cup) servings

1 (6-ounce) can tomato paste
¼ cup honey
¼ cup water
3 tablespoons apple cider vinegar
Sea salt
Freshly ground black pepper

In a small bowl, whisk the tomato paste, honey, water, and vinegar. Season with sea salt and pepper. Refrigerate for a few hours to firm up. Keep refrigerated in an airtight container for up to 1 week.

SUBSTITUTION TIP: For a vegan version, substitute molasses for the honey.

Homemade Mustard

Prep time: 5 minutes / **Total time:** 10 minutes

Despite what many people may think, mustard is really easy to make at home. It is just mustard powder, water, sea salt, vinegar, and a little pepper to create a whole lot of flavor. You can also add fresh herbs, such as dill or tarragon, if you like.

Makes: about 1½ cups;
12 (2-tablespoon) servings

1 cup ground mustard seed
1 cup water
½ cup distilled white vinegar
Sea salt
Freshly ground black pepper

1. In a small bowl, combine the ground mustard and water. Whisk well.

2. Add the vinegar. Season with sea salt and pepper. Whisk well again. Keep refrigerated in an airtight container for up to 3 months.

> VARIATION TIP: Make a whole-grain mustard by substituting a scant ½ cup of brown mustard seeds, a scant ½ cup of yellow mustard seeds, and 2 tablespoons of ground mustard seed for the 1 cup of ground mustard seed called for in the recipe.

Cucumber Relish

Prep time: 5 minutes / Total time: 10 minutes, plus 2 to 5 days to ferment

Relish is another kitchen staple usually made with sugar. There are a few companies that make relish without sugar, which is great, but they are typically overpriced. Why spend your money on higher-end relishes when you can easily make it at home? Grab some fresh cucumbers and a few other key ingredients and you are set!

Makes: 4 cups; 32 (2-tablespoon) servings

4 large cucumbers, seeds removed, diced super finely
1 cup chopped fresh dill
2 teaspoons sea salt
½ cup white wine vinegar

1. Have ready a sterilized quart-size glass jar with a lid.

2. In a medium bowl, stir together the diced cucumbers, dill, and sea salt.

3. With a wooden spoon or your clean fist, pack the cucumber mixture tightly into the jar, making sure to extract as much water as you can from the mixture.

4. Add the vinegar, leaving at least 1 inch of headroom between the liquid and the top of the jar, as the mixture will expand while fermenting. Tightly seal the jar with the lid.

5. Place the jar in a warm place for 2 to 5 days, depending on how sour you like your relish. Keep refrigerated for up to 3 months. If you see any signs of mold, discard the relish.

VARIATION TIP: Slice the cucumbers into rounds instead of dicing them and add 1 bay leaf, 1 smashed garlic clove, and 1 teaspoon of peppercorns to make pickle chips instead of relish.

Fresh Horseradish

Prep time: 5 minutes / **Total time:** 10 minutes

Horseradish is great with nearly every beef recipe in this book and is wonderful with prime rib, steak, and even pot roast. There are two types of horseradish: creamy and straight. Straight horseradish does not have any cream and it's *really* hot. Both types are usually made with sugar. My version does not have any sugar in it. Don't be afraid to make it spicy if you are into the hot stuff!

Makes: 3 cups; 24 (2-tablespoon) servings

2 cups minced peeled fresh
    horseradish root
1 cup white wine vinegar
2 tablespoons chopped garlic
1 teaspoon sea salt

In a blender, combine the horseradish, vinegar, garlic, and sea salt. If you want straight-up horseradish, use more horseradish and less liquid. If you want creamier horseradish, use more liquid. Process to your preferred consistency. It's that simple. Keep refrigerated in an airtight container for up to 3 weeks.

> **PRO TIP:** Be careful when handling fresh horseradish root. It is very strong and, when ground in a blender, gives off an intense vapor that can burn your eyes and throat. Open the blender as far as possible from your face, and resist the urge to take a big whiff!

Beet Relish

Prep time: 5 minutes / **Total time:** 10 minutes, plus 2 to 3 days to ferment

Have you ever had beet relish? It's a unique and interesting twist on traditional relish. It's tart, fruity, and has a vibrant taste. Add this to your sausage and egg recipes for guaranteed success! Making beet relish is the same as making traditional relish. The longer you let it ferment, the better the flavor will be.

Makes: about 3 cups; 6 (½-cup) servings

2 cups Japanese cucumbers, diced super finely
1 cup beet juice, strained
1 cup distilled white vinegar
1 teaspoon sea salt

1. Have ready a sterilized quart-size glass jar with a lid.

2. In a large bowl, combine the cucumbers, beet juice, vinegar, and sea salt. Stir to mix well. Transfer to the jar and tightly cover with the lid.

3. Set the jar aside to ferment for 2 to 3 days. The longer it ferments, the stronger it will taste. Keep refrigerated for 4 to 6 months, sealed.

> VARIATION TIP: For a flavor twist, add 1 pinch of celery seeds and/or fennel or caraway seeds to the mix.

Barbecue Sauce

Prep time: 5 minutes / **Cook time:** 40 minutes / **Total time:** 45 minutes

This recipe takes a little more time, but I believe it's worth it and I bet you will never go back to store-bought sauce again. You do need homemade ketchup and mustard for this recipe. I suggest making those ahead so you're ready to go.

Makes: about 4 cups;
8 (½-cup) servings

1 garlic clove, minced
2 (6-ounce) cans tomato paste
1 cup apple cider vinegar
1 cup water
½ cup Simple Ketchup (page 127)
¾ cup Homemade Mustard (page 128)
2 tablespoons coconut aminos

In a large skillet over low heat, stir together the garlic, tomato paste, vinegar, water, ketchup, mustard, and coconut aminos. Simmer for 30 to 40 minutes. Transfer to a glass jar with a lid, tightly seal, and refrigerate for up to 3 weeks.

VARIATION TIP: Make a punchier sauce by adding 1 minced onion, 1 teaspoon of paprika, a dash of ground cinnamon and cloves, and a splash of hot sauce along with the other ingredients.

Paleo Tomato Sauce

Prep time: 5 minutes / **Cook time:** 10 minutes / **Total time:** 15 minutes

We all love a good tomato sauce! A good Italian-style tomato sauce can be used in everything from meatball recipes to baked zucchini recipes—it's truly a staple sauce everyone needs. Traditional Italian sauce is made with a lot of sugar, which is unnecessary because tomatoes are naturally quite sweet. Prep this easy Paleo Tomato Sauce on a Sunday and you'll have plenty for recipes for the entire week.

Makes: about 8 cups

2 cups chopped Roma tomatoes
½ cup chicken stock
1 onion, minced
4 garlic cloves, minced
¼ cup olive oil
¼ cup fresh parsley, minced
½ teaspoon dried oregano

1. Heat the olive oil in a skillet over medium heat for about 30 seconds.

2. Add the minced onion and minced garlic to the skillet and sauté the onion and garlic for 2 to 3 minutes, or until browned.

3. Pour the chicken stock into the skillet and sauté everything together for 1 minute.

4. Add the chopped tomatoes, fresh parsley, and dried oregano, and simmer on low heat for 10 to 15 minutes, or until the sauce is nice and thick.

> **PRO TIP:** Paleo Tomato Sauce will store in the freezer in an airtight container for up to 6 months.

Citrus Vinaigrette

Prep time: 5 minutes / **Total time:** 10 minutes

Citrus vinaigrette is very versatile. There is no reason ever to buy store-bought vinaigrette because you can make it at home with the ingredients you have on your kitchen counter. As long as you have lemons or limes and fresh garlic you are good to go.

Makes: about 1½ cups; 12 (2-tablespoon) servings

1 cup EVOO
½ cup freshly squeezed lemon juice or lime juice
1 garlic clove, minced
1 tablespoon sea salt
2 tablespoons freshly ground black pepper

In a pint-size glass jar with a lid, combine the EVOO, lemon or lime juice, garlic, sea salt, and pepper. Secure the cap tightly and shake everything really well until combined. Keep refrigerated for up to 3 weeks.

> **VARIATION TIP:** This vinaigrette is super versatile. Add any number of herbs, spices, or aromatics to change the flavor profile. I like to add minced shallot, minced fresh rosemary or oregano, paprika and ground cumin, and even a dollop of Dijon mustard or honey.

Balsamic Vinaigrette

Prep time: 5 minutes / Total time: 10 minutes

Balsamic vinaigrette is a delicious homemade dressing to have on hand any time you need a quick salad dressing. You do not have to use all the fresh herbs called for if you do not want to. They add more flavor to the vinaigrette and the more you use, the more flavorful your vinaigrette will be.

Makes: about 1 cup;
8 (2-tablespoon) servings

2 tablespoons fresh rosemary leaves
2 tablespoons fresh oregano leaves
1 garlic clove, minced
¼ cup freshly squeezed lemon juice
¼ cup balsamic vinegar
½ cup EVOO

1. In a food processor, pulse the rosemary and oregano until finely minced.

2. Add the garlic. Pulse again for 30 seconds.

3. Add the lemon juice, vinegar, and EVOO. Pulse for 1 minute more until the dressing is well blended. Transfer to a glass jar with a lid, tightly seal, and refrigerate for up to 1 week.

> VARIATION TIP: Vary the flavor of this dressing by changing the herbs. Try adding or substituting fresh basil, mint, tarragon, or parsley.

Caesar Dressing

Prep time: 5 minutes / Total time: 10 minutes

If you like Caesar salad and you like the taste of anchovies, you are going to love this easy, spiced-up Paleo Caesar dressing.

Makes: about 1½ cups; 6 [¼-cup] servings

½ cup Homemade Mayonnaise [page 126]
⅓ cup EVOO
¼ cup minced anchovies
3 garlic cloves, minced
1 tablespoon Dijon mustard
1 tablespoon freshly squeezed lemon juice
Sea salt
Freshly ground black pepper

In a food processor, combine the mayonnaise, EVOO, anchovies, garlic, mustard, and lemon juice. Season with sea salt and pepper. Blend for 1 minute until smooth. Add a bit of water, if needed, to achieve the right consistency. Transfer to a glass jar with a lid, tightly seal, and refrigerate for up to 1 week.

SUBSTITUTION TIP: For a vegetarian version, leave out the anchovies and substitute ¼ cup of minced oil-cured olives to keep the salty, umami flavor.

Paleo Ranch Dressing

Prep time: 5 minutes / Total time: 5 minutes

Ranch dressing is delicious. There are no two ways about it. In fact, I've never met a person who didn't love ranch dressing. You miss ranch dressing on the Paleo diet, but not with my healthy twist on it. The fresh herbs give this a bright taste and the chives give it a nice bite.

Makes: about 1¼ cups;
7 (¼-cup) servings

1 cup Homemade Mayonnaise
   (page 126)
½ cup full-fat coconut cream
¼ cup chopped fresh parsley
¼ cup chopped fresh dill
¼ cup chopped fresh chives
1 teaspoon sea salt

In a food processor, combine the mayonnaise, coconut cream, parsley, dill, chives, and sea salt. Process until everything is well combined. Transfer to a glass jar with a lid, tightly seal, and refrigerate for up to 1 week.

VARIATION TIP: Add 1 or 2 garlic cloves along with the other ingredients, or use 1 teaspoon of garlic powder.

Easy Guacamole

Prep time: 5 minutes / **Total time:** 10 minutes

Guacamole is a staple in every diet. Well, let's be honest, if it isn't it should be. There is no "special" way to make guacamole or to name it Paleo. Just use basic, fresh, simple ingredients and you have an easy dip for all those veggies.

Makes: about 2 cups;
8 (¼-cup) servings

4 avocados, peeled, halved,
  pitted, and finely diced
1 medium red onion, finely diced
Juice of 2 limes
Juice of ½ to 1 lemon
1 tablespoon freshly ground
  black pepper
1½ teaspoons sea salt

In a food processor, combine the avocados, red onion, lime juice, lemon juice, pepper, and sea salt. Process until smooth. Refrigerate the guacamole in an airtight glass container, with a layer of water on top to keep it fresh. It will keep for a few days. Just pour off the water and stir up the guac before serving.

VARIATION TIP: If you really want to amp up your guac, add 1 teaspoon of minced garlic.

Cauliflower Tortillas

Prep time: 10 minutes / **Cook time:** 15 minutes / **Total time:** 25 minutes

Say goodbye to conventional taco shells. Make these ahead of time on your prep day for taco Tuesday any day of the week. You can even freeze them in a zip-top bag for up to 6 months. Cauliflower tortillas are a famous Paleo staple. Cauliflower is nutritionally dense and easily accessible year-round. And, although it doesn't pack a huge flavor punch, it does add a certain richness to your meals.

Makes: 8 tortillas

1 head cauliflower, cut into florets
2 large eggs
1 cup chopped fresh cilantro
4 garlic cloves
1 teaspoon paprika
Sea salt
Freshly ground black pepper

1. Preheat the oven to 400°F. Line two baking sheets with parchment paper and set aside.

2. In a blender or food processor, pulse the cauliflower until you get a texture similar to rice.

3. Add the eggs, cilantro, garlic, and paprika. Season with sea salt and pepper. Pulse for 3 minutes until combined. Scoop the mixture onto the prepared baking sheets and form it into round circles, as thick or thin as you like.

4. Bake for 15 minutes until golden brown, switching the baking sheets from top to bottom and front to back halfway through the baking time.

5. Let cool. Refrigerate in a sealed glass container for up to 5 days, or freeze.

> PRO TIP: These will hold together better if you press excess liquid out of the riced cauliflower before adding the eggs and other ingredients. To do so, scoop the riced cauliflower out of the food processor into a clean dishtowel and squeeze out as much liquid as you can. Return the cauliflower to the food processor and proceed with the recipe.

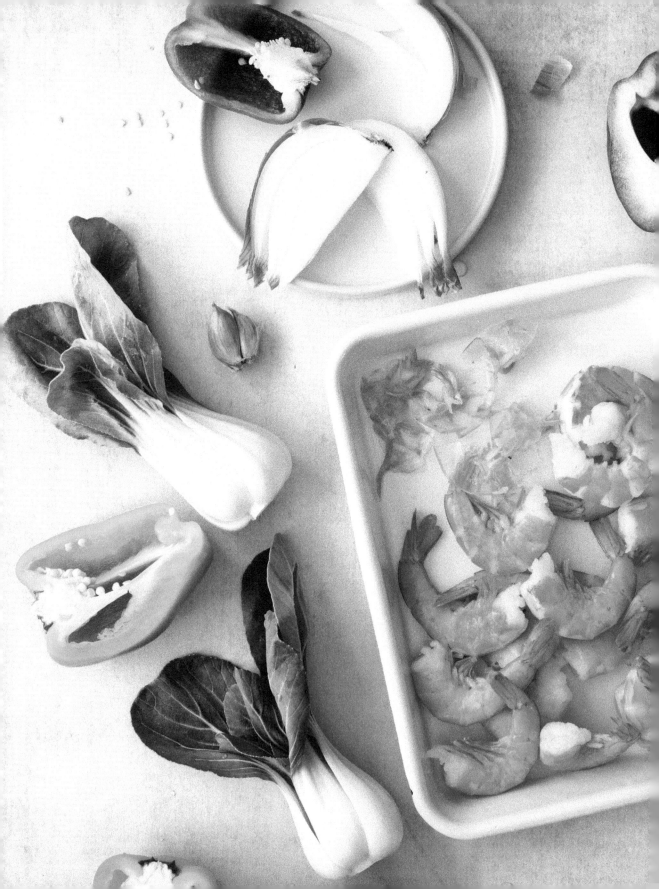

Measurement Conversions

Volume Equivalents (Liquid)

STANDARD	US STANDARD (OUNCES)	METRIC (APPROXIMATE)
2 tablespoons	1 fl. oz.	30 mL
¼ cup	2 fl. oz.	60 mL
½ cup	4 fl. oz.	120 mL
1 cup	8 fl. oz.	240 mL
1½ cups	12 fl. oz.	355 mL
2 cups or 1 pint	16 fl. oz.	475 mL
4 cups or 1 quart	32 fl. oz.	1 L
1 gallon	128 fl. oz.	4 L

Oven Temperatures

FAHRENHEIT (F)	CELSIUS (C) (APPROXIMATE)
250° F	120° C
300° F	150° C
325° F	165° C
350° F	180° C
375° F	190° C
400° F	200° C
425° F	220° C
450° F	230° C

Volume Equivalents (Dry)

STANDARD	METRIC (APPROXIMATE)
⅛ teaspoon	0.5 mL
¼ teaspoon	1 mL
½ teaspoon	2 mL
¾ teaspoon	4 mL
1 teaspoon	5 mL
1 tablespoon	15 mL
¼ cup	59 mL
⅓ cup	79 mL
½ cup	118 mL
⅔ cup	156 mL
¾ cup	177 mL
1 cup	235 mL
2 cups or 1 pint	475 mL
3 cups	700 mL
4 cups or 1 quart	1 L

Weight Equivalents

STANDARD	METRIC (APPROXIMATE)
½ ounce	15 g
1 ounce	30 g
2 ounces	60 g
4 ounces	115 g
8 ounces	225 g
12 ounces	340 g
16 ounces or 1 pound	455 g

The Dirty Dozen & the Clean Fifteen™

A nonprofit environmental watchdog organization called Environmental Working Group (EWG) looks at data supplied by the U.S. Department of Agriculture (USDA) and the Food and Drug Administration (FDA) about pesticide residues. Each year it compiles a list of the best and worst pesticide loads found in commercial crops. You can use these lists to decide which fruits and vegetables to buy organic to minimize your exposure to pesticides and which produce is considered safe enough to buy conventionally. This does not mean they are pesticide-free, though, so wash these fruits and vegetables thoroughly.

Clean Fifteen™

- asparagus
- avocados
- broccoli
- cabbages
- cantaloupes
- cauliflower
- eggplants
- honeydew melons
- kiwis
- mangos
- onions
- papayas
- pineapples
- sweet corn
- sweet peas (frozen)

Dirty Dozen™

- apples
- celery
- cherries
- grapes
- nectarines
- peaches
- pears
- potatoes
- spinach
- strawberries
- sweet bell peppers
- tomatoes

Additionally, nearly three-quarters of hot pepper samples contained pesticide residues

Recipe Type Index

Recipe Index

Index

About the Author

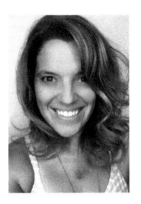

Genevieve Jerome is a full-time blogger and health and wellness expert. At FittyFoodlicious.com she writes about healing our bodies with food, creates real-food recipes, and talks openly about mental health, hormones, and how radical self-love can change the world. When she's not writing or creating new recipes, you can find her hitting the running trails with her dogs, kayaking, rock climbing, traveling, chasing the sun with her lens, and drinking copious amounts of coffee and sparkling water. Genevieve resides in Northern California with her husband and family.

CPSIA information can be obtained
at www.ICGtesting.com
Printed in the USA
BVHW05s0117151018
530129BV00001B/1/P

9 781641 521116